Grow Young

Integrate Healthy & Balanced Changes Into Your Life

Victory Assaf
only U can change U

Notice

This book is not intended to replace recommendations or advice from physicians or other healthcare providers. It is rather oriented to help you dive deep into your life and make changes that you feel will have a positive impact on your lifestyle. If you suspect you have a medical problem, we urge you to seek medical attention from a competent healthcare provider.

To contact the author, visit www.zestylifestylez.com

Victory Assaf
Lifestyle Consultant / Motivational Speaker / Author

Contents

Acknowledgments

I would love to express gratitude to all the people I have met throughout my life and who have inspired me and made me the person I am today. Thank you dearly for being such inspirational and internally beautiful people.

I would love to cordially thank:

My sweet **Dad** and my world **Mum**, loved you yesterday, love you today and will love you forever.I am blessed to have you in my life.

My lovely brother **Tony** and his beautiful motivating wife **Ruba**, for your continuous support and care all the way, I love you guys.

Francois Saade, President of the Lebanese Judo Federation and Owner of Bouddha Sports City, for your continuos support and motivation throughout the 20 years.

Harry Atallah, the dearest cousin in the whole world, for your eccentric creativity, I made sure that you will be the only person who shall design my book. Keep soaring lovely cousin.

Joshua Rosenthal, Founder of the Institute for Integrative Nutrition, for your creative initiatives and continuous motivation which are the reasons behind my writing. Keep Shining.

Lindsey Smith, Author and Motivational Speaker, for your motivation, passion and positive vibes which have been felt all the way from New York to Lebanon.

Darren Danks, Holistic Health Coach, for sharing with me your inspiring experience. Good luck star.

Dr. Mostafa M. Shaheen, (M.B.B.CH.,MBA,CFE,PMP) for your time and precious involvement; for your medical contribution and advice which helped in providing my book with accurate medical details.

All my friends who have supported me throughout my journey. It's a nice feeling to have sisters but it's a lavish feeling to find best friends and consider them the sisters I've never had.

And special thanks go to:

Sandy Savo, for your positive presence next to me throughout my book journey which made a big difference; for your support and genuine friendship.

Nadine Waked, for the beautiful 20 years of memorable experiences and fun adventures.

Chantal Melki Chalhoub, for the 18 years of positive and inspiring vibes that you have always extended to me.

Viviane Maalouf, for your lovely spirit and beautiful soul. I cherish our unforgettable memories in Qatar.

Last but not least, **Roula Barrak Hanna**, my beautiful editor, for all your efforts and time; for your contribution to my book with your positive energy and valuable input.

For whoever will choose to have my book among their book collections.

Introduction

To have selected my book, means the title, **Grow Young**, has triggered your curiosity and grabbed your attention, and I am happy it did because it's all in here. This book is all about initiating a beautiful relationship between yourself, your body and your life so that you arrive to lead a healthy and positive lifestyle.

Whether you're a female or male; whether you're single or married; the mission of my book is to create an energetic buzz and guide you to find the lifestyle choices that best support you. It will also help you to make gradual, lifelong changes that enable you to reach your current and future health goals in a way that is flexible, fun and rewarding.

I consider my life to be a book I need to fill with unlimited interesting chapters.
"Book of Life"

Hence, this book in particular is filled with chapters that highlight 36 years of multiple experiences that have challenged me and forged me into becoming the person I am today. I love to face my challenges and live new experiences to be able to fill the rest of my chapters with memorable stories and to be able to have a beautiful ending to my book...**My Life.**

Everyone is entitled to write this "book of life "one day. In fact, this is possible since the material lies within each one of us. This latter is summed up in the challenges we encounter and experiences we live throughout any and each stage of our life. Take good care of your mind, body and soul, and you will enjoy facing your challenges. Some people face their challenges and yet live with them and others just survive them.

The people who decide to survive their challenges are unfortunately the ones that lead boring lives. They are the ones that fear to stumble upon any change. They are the ones that lack self-confidence. They are rooted in motionlessness like a tree which is firmly planted and unyielding to any wind.

On the other hand, those who decide to face their challenges and live them as well are the ones leading adventurous and exciting lives. They embrace the changes lovingly and happily. Hence, they enjoy themselves, and therefore are the ones who lead healthy lifestyles.

What is a Healthy Lifestyle?

Despite the fact that everyone has a self-tailored lifestyle, we sometimes envy others for their way of living and we sometimes pity them. But in reality, it is important to note that there is no such thing as right to envy, or wrong to pity. It is all about our perception of things, incidents, people...**LIFE.**

To start, a lifestyle mirrors what is within each person. It reflects the first day you were born, the first breath, the first drinks. It also reflects your eating habits, movements, parents, family, neighbors, beliefs, religion, traditions, hobbies, intensions, intuitions, puberty, education, friends, career, colleagues, intimate relationships, kids, strangers and community. A Lifestyle is **U, Your Body and Life.**

To continue, we all equally receive 6 essential gifts when we are born. Even though we are appreciative of some of these gifts, we surely dislike others. These 6 essential gifts are as follows: our body, name, parents, relatives, nationality and religion.

We don't choose any of them. It is like the Universe has conspired to impose them on us. Had we been lucky, we would have got gifts that we will always love. However, if that was not the case, we will definitely be compelled to find the necessary means to live with our undesired inheritance.

It is for those particular reasons that we come across many people who are content with what they have got and many others who keep complaining and suffering from their body, their name, their mother, their father, their relatives, their nationality and their religion till the last day of their lives.

And there are those people who although do not like some of their life's gifts, they positively try to either accept them or change them throughout their life.

The choice is thus yours. You either decide to:

Love what you have received, enjoy them and be happy;
Change some of them, accept the rest and be happy;
Learn to accept the ones you don't love and live happily; or
Survive the ones you don't love and live unhappily and in denial.

After-all, the decision is in your hand. You were born a hero. You defeated trillions of sperms to win this life. Appreciate it and enjoy a healthy living.

Conscious of the importance of healthy living and filled to the brim with the passion of motivating people into leading healthy lifestyles, I have decided to write my first book and fill it not only with catchy or beautiful words but also with motivating stories that I have personally experienced. Therefore, I had to go 36 years back and jot down my memorable challenges and experiences to create my motivational chapters for people to read, enjoy and become inspired.

In my book, I will take you through my healthy transformations and zesty lifestyle. I will share with you the importance of healthy eating and how I love to maintain regular exercise. I will also take you into my positive thinking, shed light on the need to have self-love, explain how to accept others, and many other tips. I will give you access to few of my motivational and funny stories that hopefully will pave your way to discover your inner blessings.

OneBody…
One Life …
One U

Chapter One

. My Life and I

My name is Victory Assaf, a name I admire. I was born in Lebanon to an adorable family, a Lebanese father "Pierre" and an Armenian mother "Maryette". I have one brother "Tony".

I was lucky to have parents who have oriented my brother and me to practicing sports since I was 5 years old. At first, they registered my brother in Judo classes and me in Ballet classes. Nevertheless, as I periodically used to accompany my mum to pick my brother up from his class, I fell in love with Judo and I had kept on practicing this sport until I became 25 and received my 2nd Dan Black Belt.

Throughout these years, I competed in Judo tournaments around the Globe winning local and International recognitions. I was the Lebanese Judo champion for 20 years. I was also awarded other recognitions such as International, Francophone and Pan Arab champion.

My brother likewise had won the 3rd position for the world's Judo Championship in Spain but he unfortunately stopped his Judo practices due to a serious arm injury and yet, instead of quitting sports entirely and living with his injury, he had alternatively chosen football and basketball.

My first 25 years were spent studying, working and practicing all kinds of sports in Lebanon.

During my university studies I was literally leading a very active and busy life, from managing my studies, to working in 4 schools as a part time Athletic Director and a Judo Coach, to attending my Judo trainings at night. Moreover, at the weekends I used to organize skiing and ice-skating classes for my students. Despite all the hustle, I loved sharing energy with my students and taught them how to enjoy sports and be active.

Being a female Judo athlete, I was invited to many TV and Radio programs and was also interviewed by local and international magazines to talk about my achievements and motivate people, especially ladies and kids, to do sports. I also used to present Judo tournaments that were broadcasted live on some famous Lebanese TV channels. This basically made me somehow a known athlete in Lebanon.

After I graduated from the Lebanese International Faculty of Science and received a BA in Political Science, my corporate world challenges started. Nevertheless, my choice to study Political Science was mainly to satisfy my mother's passion who always wanted me to work in the diplomatic sector.

Hence, i was offered 2 full time positions, one in the Political Sector and one in Hospitality. So following my passion, you can surely guess that I joined one of the leading hotels in Lebanon to manage its newly launched wellness facility, and my leisure career has kicked off from that moment. I started to join international wellness institutions to have an in-depth knowledge of this particular field.

After excelling at my work for 2 years, I decided to leave Lebanon and travel abroad to experience new personal as well as career challenges.

I have never been the routine or conventional girl. I loved changes and new challenges were my best friend. My next destinations were United Arab of Emirates, then Yemen and finally Qatar. Throughout my 12 years in the corporate world I have developed and managed luxurious Wellness and Leisure projects.

In Qatar I joined one of the biggest luxurious Qatari companies where I worked for almost 5 years. I was enjoying every bit of it until I started to wonder what is really missing in my life. I mulled over whether it is the time for a new challenge or whether I should make a drastic change.

Soon a vivid new light was shed by me intuitively. I felt the need for a break from work and the need to spend quality time with the ones I love back home. I needed to take care of myself. I needed to start doing something different, something which can help me share my passion in a vast way that aims at raising healthy awareness to communities.

I wanted to find creative ways to keep motivating people and spread my passion among everyone, aiming to transform their lifestyle to a healthy one. It was the time to pull myself out from my comfort zone. My instinct led the way, and helped me realize that whenever my work and life enter the viscous circle of routine I lose interest and I start looking for new challenges to boost my life.

In a rush, I packed my things, thanked my employers and colleagues, bid farewell to Qatar and moved back to Lebanon where I embraced my family again, enjoyed quality time with my parents, my close friends and my tiny Yorkshire dog " Youpi". I can't move on with this topic without highlighting the great career and personal development that I have gained over the past 5 years in this luxurious Qatari company where my relationship with the owners and their beautiful families was very special as till date I consider them as my sincere family in Qatar.

You might be astounded by my rapid shift. The thing is people especially single ones who live abroad always fear the moment when their parents might leave this world. This is exactly how I used to feel. For this reason, I wanted to spend more time with my family, enjoy their growing "Young" process and motivate them for healthy living.

I deeply believe that my instability and love of life are the reasons behind my active life. I have billions of stories to share with you, stay tuned.

My transformation started here. After I resigned, I started to search for new ways to boost my passion and dive in its ocean. I signed up for the Institute for Integrative Nutrition (IIN), known to be the largest Nutrition and Health Coaching school in the world based in New York. My health journey kicked off from this school.

Throughout my years, I've read lots of motivational, inspiring and lifestyle oriented books. I even used to motivate my friends to start reading the books that had enthused me and taught me to always stay grateful and to live abundantly. I always felt the passion to write myself my own personalized book one day to touch people's hearts easily.

Like I said, I always had the dream to write a book. I always wanted to share my experience and healthy lifestyle with others, until the opportunity struck me deep.Here I am sharing with you my first book in which I tried to inject all the necessary information that I have learnt and experienced to help you look deep into yourself and pamper your soul and body in the right and healthy way for a happy life.

**"The mission of my book
is to create an energetic
buzz and spread healthy
and positive vibes in
every house and in every
individual's life..."**

Chapter Two

No Diet Lasts, Only a Healthy Way of Eating

During my childhood and teenage years, I followed numerous weight management programs set to me by nutritionists and dietitians. Each specialist I met recommended a different diet. I read billions of diet and nutrition books and once again each book highlighted specific diets and new methods of losing weight.

I used to watch many health-oriented programs on TV as well, but nothing caught my attention. At the end, they all failed to meet my expectations and very soon I found myself bored from the diet system which led me to strongly believe that there is no such thing as diet; however, there is only a healthy way of eating.

Growing up, I was always obedient and ate what mum cooked trusting her and trusting that it's the right and healthy choice of food. Hence, I grew up eating almost everything. Sweets were my weakness. For instance, I abundantly ate chocolate, biscuits and ice cream. I just love them!!! Moreover, being a Judo athlete, I used to have a number of weight challenges during some tournaments as I had to put on and lose weight constantly to be able to take part in different categories during the tournaments. Putting on weight was way easier than losing it. I am sure many agree with me on this.

I sometimes used to eat a full pack of chips or chocolate at night thinking that my body needed it. And the next day when I felt down and not energetic, I used to think it's due to the weather. I never thought that my body was communicating with me. I was totally disconnected from my body and always favored restaurants food. Most of the time, I was on a YOYO diet. For example, I used to cut out sweets and bread and eat grilled food all the time. Almost every Monday, I used to set a goal to start a new diet. I am sure many people follow this trend too. Unfortunately, I never really succeeded in finding a balanced diet and this has affected my skin elasticity in the long run.

After losing hope from all the weight management programs and recommendations and rejecting the existence of the word diet, I started to design my own way of eating. It meant eating low fat based dairies, grilled meat, chicken and fish, salads and fruits and whatever I thought was healthy and contained low amount of calories.

Leading a busy, active career and a sporty life pushed me away from the kitchen and I grew up not having a tiny idea on how to prepare a simple meal not even a salad or a boiled egg. The kitchen was a grey area for me. As a matter of fact, when I started my career abroad, I lived most of my time in hotels and when I rented apartments I used not to care much about the kitchen. While in hotels, the food was of course prepared by the chefs.

Again I didn't have the urge to learn cooking. As for my apartments, I didn't even have a kitchen set up neither did I opt to bringing a small oven. I used only to enter the kitchen to drink water or turn on the washing machine, nothing more and nothing less. However, when my friends and I used to plan lunch or dinner at their place, I always offered to do the dishes as I enjoy it and was also good at it. And guess what? Sometimes, at some gatherings, I even offered to wash vegetables and squeeze lemons to feel a bit involved in the cooking process.

I have spent 36 years of my life eating a balanced quantity of processed food, refined sugar, all kinds of sweets, low fat dairies, processed meat, white bread, wheat flour, etc. Most of the time, I had lunch and dinner in the restaurants. My breakfast was on the other hand at home as I used to have fruits or yogurt. And whenever a cooking program or conversation started in a social gathering or on the telly, I used to tune out and surf my phone to chat and enjoy other different topics.

It's worth mentioning that I am neither fond of drinking coffee nor of smoking. I am not even an alcohol fan, but very occasionally I drink wine. And yet, throughout this period, I always struggled to lose my 5 extra kg but unfortunately I didn't know how. I was still sometimes losing a few kg and other times putting them on back quickly. I was exercising almost daily for a minimum of 2 hours burning around 800 calories but I still had a few kg that were stuck without any plans to leave me. It was weird. "I am an athlete who exercises regularly and I eat healthy food, then why am I not reaching the weight and the figure I long for?" I kept wondering for years...

One day and during the preparation of my first Triathlon race (an athletic contest consisting of three different events, typically swimming, cycling, and long-distance running), I realized my moves were quite heavy and I was low on energy. I felt something was going wrong every time I pushed myself hard during the training.

Only after this incident did I decided to really listen to my body and look into the right ways to lose weight and maintain a good athletic figure. And since then I've stopped believing in diets and because over the years I have tried all the ways to lose weight and nothing was fruitful, this time I decided to invest more time in examining my body and making it a food testing field.

I started to cut out some kinds of foods and increase other kinds. For example, I'd cut out sugar for a week then cut out dairies and bread for the other week. This went on for a couple of weeks during which I also cut out meat for a week and on all kinds of sweets for the subsequent week and so on. I was still exercising while trying these dieting techniques.

Surprisingly, my body felt satisfied, my moves became lighter and swifter, and I felt more energetic when I cut out the red meat and refined sugar. I, henceforth, managed to record good results in the triathlon. As of that moment, I decided to cut out red meat and become partially vegetarian. This meant to continue eating limited portions of chicken and fish.

Now and after undergoing this change I strongly believe we can always alter the food pattern we are used to. We simply need to talk and listen to our bodies. Our body is perfectly designed. We even have a built in alarm system which we need to always listen to. Our body is always in constant change. It gets affected by the level of exercise, by some habits and by environmental changes. Therefore, we should always cope with any change and be experts in reading the signs our bodies display.

During my studies, I learnt to listen more to my body. I got down to work and began to test my body's reaction to the intake of some foods and to the cutting out on others. I started cooking and preparing my own healthy meals and inviting my friends to share this fulfilling and joyful transformation with me.I learnt about food and how it is created behind the white doors. I also learnt about the packaging system and the different means by which any type of food is imported to us.

I learnt how badly I used to eat thinking low fat or processed food with low calories is healthy. I learnt that my body was resisting or more likely refusing many kinds of foods especially the ones prepared in the restaurants, because although they smell nice, they include many ingredients that are processed and full of refined sugar.

I started to love cooking. Who could have imagined me cooking?? I started to enjoy food shopping, reading labels and checking every ingredient I am fueling my body with. I started to examine what people are putting in their supermarket trolleys and what they are feeding their kids with.

Many times I felt sick and annoyed while watching those parents' trolleys getting filled with chips, chocolate, canned drinks and food and processed meat and food. Literally all sorts of junk food went into their trolleys. What is more, I learnt how to appreciate my mum's food more and feel her positivity and love in every meal she's prepared. I shared with her healthy tips so she could incorporate them in her traditional Lebanese and Armenian dishes.

Finally I became a food inspector, someone who wants to invest her time into learning more about food and protecting her system from unnecessary junk processed foods. You eat junk, you feel junk.I started to look for nutrients in everything I ate . I fell in love with vegetables and all sorts of fruits, green smoothies and all types of fresh juices became my daily breakfast and dinner. As for my energy snacks, well, I savored on raw nuts, almonds and cashews.

I started to chew better, to enjoy my meals more and to relish the flow of food in my digestive system. At last, I have started to enjoy listening to my body. However, I didn't stop there. I got a food note book on which I wrote for few months what I was eating and how I felt as a result afterwards throughout the day. This helped me to examine the food reaction in my system and learn which type of food my body is enjoying more and which food combination is good to my system.

Much to my good fortune, I now know that eating fruits straight after my meals causes me bloating. Moreover, the low energy I used to feel when I exercised heavily was because of the red meat I ate. In addition to that, I know now that if I eat sweets or bread or any kind of refined sugar my body will crave more sugar and food throughout the day. I henceforth eliminated a few types of food and introduced other new types to my system until I felt balanced and in tight relationship with my body.

Of course, experiencing the suitable types of food will never stop because our bodies keep on changing with time and age. Therefore and at all times, all we need to do is to carefully listen to the signs our body is exhibiting.

Now food shopping became my hobby. At first and for a couple of times, I was a bit confused. There are billion brands on the shelves. Plus, I had no clue which one is good for cooking because previously I used to shop for chocolate, chips, canned food, low fat dairies and very limited quantities of fruits and vegetables.

In parallel with this I started to invest my time in reading labels. I used to spend 2 to 3 hours in the supermarket reading every label of the food I was choosing for my system. I needed to learn what healthy benefits each type of food had to offer me. Reading the labels once and thoroughly meant the food could go inside my trolley. I started enjoying cleaning and washing every item I bought. As a matter of fact, I don't put any item in the fridge without making sure it is clean and well stored.

Major transformations hit my life. I subsequently changed from being the over busy career girl who enjoys restaurant food because she doesn't have the least idea about cooking into a mature woman who cooks, appreciates her body and feeds it with all healthy nutrients.

❝ Food shopping becomes healthy when you know the good nutrients & you start reading labels. ❞

Chapter Three

■ Different Body / Food / Medicine

Dieting... A constant nightmare

Nowadays, all we read about in the magazines, hear from different people, watch on TV or are advised with during nutritional consultations is centered on the different diets necessary for a healthier body as well as healthy eating recommendations. Some say breakfast is good, others say it's not. Some say don't drink lots of water, others say it is very healthy. Some say don't eat red meat, others say it's the best source of protein. Some recommend a vegan diet (no consumption of animal product), others promote a vegetarian diet (no consumption of red meat, only white meat) and the list goes on.

Throughout their lives, many people went on many diets such as DNA Diet, Macrobiotics, Paleo, Atkins, 9/10 Theory, South Beach, Vegetarian, Vegan, The Zone, Sally Fallon, Water Price diet, etc. They followed these diets for a certain period of time and then got bored and moved back to the bad eating habits once again.

In reality, the majority of people get lost when it comes to choosing the suitable diet. Many spend most of their lives moving from one nutritionist to another or spending money on weight loss pills, drinks and shakes. Unfortunately, many of these people don't succeed in satisfying their needs and achieving their weight management goals.

My Body and I Reunited

As I mentioned in the previous chapter, I did not use to care what food is good for me. I was totally ignoring my body. I fueled it with food that I read about or was advised to try by friends or nutritionists and that was entitled to be good and healthy. I literally tried most of my friends' diets, but nothing really worked. I always used to relate my discomfort to external factors such as the weather, work stress, homesickness, spoiled food and other things, but never really bothered to disconnect from the whole world and be attentive to listening to and appreciating the closest thing to me, **My Body.**

Due to the fact that I never invested my time into thoroughly understanding my body, I suffered from many discomforts. Many times I had skin irritations, bloating, low energy levels, mood swings, disturbed sleep, dehydration, etc. Nevertheless, I was never really interested in knowing the reason behind these reactions, because of my hectic life at work and my involvement in many sports and social activities.

Luckily, my body has been loyal to me since the day I was born despite my nonchalance. It will also stay connected to me until the last day of my life. Yet, and evidently enough, the only communication tools my body is capable of using to communicate with me is its alarm that sends signs highlighting the physical and mental comforts or discomforts.

Fortunately now, at the age of 36, I learnt one of the most insightful things in life. I learnt how to listen to my body, how to communicate with my internal system and how to appreciate its involuntary functions. I finally learnt how to Love and be Loyal to my body.

However, and unfortunately this is not the case for many people. There is for instance an interesting global trend which goes without saying that when one person had a successful result in losing weight by following a specific diet, all his/her friends want to follow the same diet. Obviously and sadly not all of them will lose weight.

For example, I had a client that had lost 11 kg in 2 months following a specific diet recommended by one of my nutritionists and a fitness program designed by one of my personal trainers. Around 10 of his friends joined the program afterwards. Alas, none of them got the same result. As a matter of fact, few got demotivated and left the program midway; others lost 2 to 3 kg in around maybe 2 months and were surely unhappy. The reason behind this disparity is that they all lead different lifestyles. They were all committed differently to the program. As an example, some cheated in some foods, others exercised less and others followed exactly all the instructions but their bodies failed to respond in the same way.

Lesson learned: Different bodies need different personalized programs...

Bio Individuality & Functional Medicine

To broaden my knowledge, I enrolled at the IIN where I was offered training in more than one hundred dietary theories, and studied a variety of practical lifestyle techniques and innovative coaching methods with some of the world's top health and wellness experts. My teachers included Dr. Andrew Weil, Director of the Arizona Center for Integrative Medicine; Dr. Deepak Chopra, leader in the field of mind-body medicine; Dr. David Katz, Director of Yale University's Prevention Research Center; Dr. Walter Willett, Chair of Nutrition at Harvard University and many other leading researchers and nutrition authorities.

My education has equipped me with extensive knowledge in holistic nutrition, health coaching, and preventive health. For instance, I screened out adequate dieting techniques more and I learnt that there is no diet that lasts. Only healthy eating lives longer. I learnt about Bio Individuality and that each body reacts differently to the same food. I also learnt about Functional Medicine and that everybody reacts differently to medication and treatments.

Bio Individuality

I have learnt plenty of things from Joshua Rosenthal, founder of the Institute for Integrative Nutrition. He's taught me that there's no one-size fits all diet. Each person is a unique individual with highly individualized nutritional requirements.

Personal differences in anatomy, metabolism, body composition and cell structure, all influence your overall health in addition to the foods that must equip your body with the necessary vitamins to make you healthier .That's why no single way of eating works for everyone. The food that is perfect for your unique body, age and lifestyle may make another person gain weight and feel lethargic.

That is why, men eat differently than women; children eat differently than adults and we all have very different preferences. Our personal tastes and inclinations, natural shapes and sizes, blood types, metabolic rates and genetic backgrounds influence what foods will and won't nourish us.

In 1956 Roger Williams published "Biochemical Individuality" asserting that individuality permeates each part of the human body. This book explained how personal differences in anatomy, metabolism and composition of bodily fluids and cell structure influence your overall health. Each person William wrote, has genetically determined and highly individualistic nutrition requirements.

What Did Your Ancestors Eat?

One of the major factors shaping bio individuality is ancestry. If many generations of your ancestors from Scandinavia were accustomed to eating dairy on a daily basis, it's natural that your body will be able to assimilate dairy foods.
By contrast, most traditional African communities did not regularly consume milk products, so it makes sense that a lot of people of African descent today are lactose intolerant.

Your Metabolic Effect

Another aspect of Bio Individuality is metabolism, or the rate at which you convert food into energy. You may recall that as a teenager you could wolf down a burger, fries, a milkshake and ice cream all in one meal without any indigestion or tightening of your jeans. That's because young people have fast metabolic rates and burn calories more quickly than adults. Even adults have different types of metabolic activity that all require varying proportions of carbohydrates, proteins, and fats. Hence, knowing what you metabolize best will help you choose foods that support your own body.

Note also that our metabolism is highly and mostly affected by age, exercise patterns and by the food we eat especially when we sometimes suffer from nutritional deficiencies. That is why since we cannot control the aging process, we need to manage to keep our metabolism in control through eating the right nutrients, exercising regularly, catching up with 7 to 8 hours of sleep per day and leading a positive lifestyle.

I, for example, used to eat the same food and practice the same kind of exercise for years. Nevertheless, I realized that I started to put on weight. When I checked with my Dr., he explained to me the fact that the metabolic rate changes with years. Therefore, I need to exercise more to burn the same amount of food I used to eat when I was younger, or to decrease the amount of food if I want to stick to my routine exercise.

These are just a few truths of the factors that influence what foods will and won't nourish you. Ultimately, one person's food may be another person's poison and that is why fad diets don't work in the long run. You need to find the kind of foods that work best for you.

Indeed, we all know people who can eat processed carbohydrates such as bread and pasta and stay very thin while others gain weight on such a diet. It's not because carbohydrates are bad or our body isn't as healthy as theirs. It just shows that all people metabolize these types of food differently. I personally do better on a high-carb diet with lots of fruits and vegetables, some beans and fish.

People are different, thus initiating a close relationship and getting to know your own body is an essential step to stay healthy. People can be divided into three general types of metabolic rates. Check which one you think you are and take appropriate measures.

1. Fast Burners: Fast burners or protein type tend to be frequently hungry and crave fatty, salty foods and do not do well on high carbohydrates or vegetarian type diets. Their bodies burn carbohydrates too quickly and a higher protein intake helps slow down their metabolism.

2. Slow Burners: Slow burners or carb types generally have relatively weak appetites, a high tolerance for sweets and problems with weight control. They require a higher percentage of carbohydrates to give them energy to speed up their metabolism.

3. Mixed Types: Generally have average appetites and moderate cravings for sweets and starchy foods. For them the ideal diet is a balanced combination of protein and carbohydrates.

Now that you know to which type of metabolic activity your body belongs, it is very important to measure your Basal Metabolic Rate (BMR). BMR is an estimate of how many calories you'd burn if you were to do nothing but rest for 24 hours. It represents the minimum amount of energy needed to keep your body functioning, including breathing and keeping your heart beating.

Having said that, many doctors and nutritionists believe that it's "calories in" and "calories out" that matter in terms of weight loss. Dr. Mark Hyman, MD and Chairman for the Institute for Functional Medicine, clearly explains that weight loss is about the quality of the calories you eat. If you consume junk you are going to get a junky metabolism, and if you eat good food you are going to get a good metabolism.

You should henceforth eat a good quality of protein (fish, chicken eggs, nuts, seeds and beans), a good quality of carbohydrates (fruits and vegetables) and a good quality of fats (avocado, almonds and olive oil).

You can measure your BMR through the most commonly used formula, the Mifflin - St Jeer equation.

a. For Men:
BMR = (10 x weight) + (6.25 x height) – (5 x age) + 5
Example: The BMR of a 40 – year-old man who weighs 85kg and is 190 cm tall is 1842.5 calories per day.
(10 x 85kg) + (6.25 x 190 cm) – (5 x 40y) + 5 = 1842.5

b. For Women:
BMR = (10 x weight) + (6.25 x height) – (5 x age) – 161
Example: My BMR is around 1371.5 calories per day (Age-36; Weight - 65; Height –170cm)
(10 x 65 kg) + (6.25 x 170 cm) – (5 x 36) – 161 = 1371.5 calories per day.

Finally, you can relate now why we enroll in weight management programs and we fail to continue as we will be advised with food that isn't compatible with our bodies. We therefore keep on craving wrong foods until we fail to manage our own weight and unfortunately we soon get bored and return to our unhealthy eating habits.

My advice for you is to eat the good food in balanced quantities and if you lose weight quickly, be happy about it as this will give you a good boost. You will definitely be proud of yourself, and feel more energetic, inspired and motivated. In fact, this happened to me when I started eating the right food and lost weight quickly and never put it back. I didn't starve myself because I've learned that even if we can arrive to lose weight by starving ourselves we'll put it back faster and at a larger scale, as our body is programmed to fight against starvation.

So the best way to lose weight is not to watch for calories, carbs, fat, or starve yourself but to eat the right type of food that will assist you to lose weight or keep your weight in balance.

Your Blood Type Effects

Many people don't know what their blood types are unless they have donated blood or received a blood transfusion. Thus it is not quite surprising that many people have no clue that there is a strong relationship between their blood type and the food they eat. I've learnt many important things form IIN concerning blood types and would therefore gladly love to share them with you. Did you for instance know that the four blood types (A, B, AB, O) have evolved for thousands of years and offer insight into what foods work best in your body? As a matter of fact, each type can be traced to a certain period of human history with distinct differences in diet, culture and social conditions. Moreover, each blood type has developed particular strengths and limitations and knowing them can influence your health. Below are details about your blood type in addition to some recommendations that can help you become more knowledgeable of your body.

Type A

Food and Allergies: People like me belonging to type "A" feel energized after eating vegetables and fruits.

Strength: They adapt well to changes in diets and the environment. They show little need for animal foods and their immune system preserves and metabolizes nutrients more easily.

Weakness: They have got a sensitive digestive tract and a vulnerable immune system which is prone to microbial invasion.

Character: They are cooperative, sensitive, orderly, settled and cultivated.

Sports: They are keen on calming and centering exercises, such as yoga and tae-chi.

Health Risks: They are subject to heart diseases, cancer, anemia, liver and gallbladder disorders and type 1 diabetes.

Diet: It is recommended that they reduce wheat, Lima beans, kidney beans, meat and dairy; and increase fruits, vegetable oil, soy foods, vegetables and pineapple.

Type B

Food and Allergies: Type "B" people are more likely to naturally tolerate dairy products.

Strength: They possess a strong immune system, they've a versatile adaption to changes in diets and the environment and have a strong nervous system.

Weakness: They have no natural weakness and yet, their autoimmune system has a tendency to breakdown and thus they have a tendency to catch viruses.

Character: They are likely to be nomadic, flexible and creative.

Sports: They are keen on sports that require moderate physical strength and a mental balance such as biking, tennis and swimming.

Health Risks: They are prone to type 1 diabetes, chronic fatigue syndrome, auto immune disorders and multiple sclerosis.

Diet: It is advisable that they reduce wheat, lentils, peanuts, sesame seeds, buckwheat and increase greens, eggs, venison, liver and licorice tea.

Type AB

Food and Allergies: Type "AB" is the most newly evolved blood type.

Strength: We tend to feel that people who have the blood type "AB" are designed for modern life. They've got a rugged immune system. They profit from the combined benefits of Type A and Type B. They are the most adaptable and can absorb information quickly.

Weakness: They can suffer from having a sensitive digestive tract. They can have an over-tolerant immune system that allows microbial invasions and they can have trouble feeling understood by the society.

Character: They are likely to be rare, enigmatic, mysterious, highly sensitive.

Sports: They can prefer calming and centering exercises such as yoga or tai-chi in addition to moderate physical exercises such as hiking, cycling and tennis.

Health Risks: They may suffer from heart diseases, cancer or anemia.

Diet: It is advisable that they reduce red meat, kidney beans, Lima beans, seeds, corn, buckwheat and increase tofu, seafood, high-quality dairy products, greens, kelp and pineapple.

Type O

Food and Allergies: Many people belonging to the type "O" feel energized by eating meat because they have strong enzymes to digest meat. They like high protein food, vegetables and fruits.

Strength: They drive benefits from their strong hard digesting tract, strong immune system, natural defenses against infections, efficient metabolism, shorter small intestines and finally a less chance to get cancer.

Weakness: They can exhibit a low tolerance for new diets and new environments. Their immune system can be over-active and attack itself. Finally the baked goods may make them feel inexplicably tired.

Character: They are often strong, self-reliant, goal-oriented and can be described as hunters and leaders.

Sports: They enjoy the over intense physical exercise such as running, aerobics, contact sports, martial arts and power yoga.

Health Risks: They may be subject to having low levels of thyroid, inflammation, arthritis, blood clotting disorders and lastly ulcers because they get overly acidic.

Diet: It is recommended that they reduce wheat/corn, baked goods, kidney beans, lentils, cauliflower and increase kelp, seafood, salt, liver/red meat, kale, spinach, broccoli and pineapple.

Once again you need to remember that our personal tastes and preferences, natural shapes and sizes, metabolic rates and genetic background influence what food will and won't nourish us. Thus, my general recommendations to you are to increase your fresh vegetables and fruits intake. Try to find local farmers who sell pure organic vegetables, fruits and products. If you can't find a local farmer then it is fine to invest in good quality vegetables and fruits for you and your family. You have one body, don't only cover it with expensive brands from outside but also make sure you feed it with quality foods that will assist your external look.

Functional Medicine

What is FM?

Dr. Mark Hyman, MD and Chairman of the Institute for Functional Medicine, is one of the Drs. who's inspired me a lot.

FM addresses the underlying causes of disease, using a systems-oriented approach and engaging both patient and practitioner in a therapeutic partnership. It is an evolution in the practice of medicine that better addresses the healthcare needs of the 21st century. By shifting the traditional disease-centered focus of medical practice to a more patient-centered approach, Functional Medicine addresses the whole person, not just an isolated set of symptoms.

Functional Medicine practitioners spend time with their patients, listening to their histories and looking at the interactions among genetic, environmental, and lifestyle factors that can influence long-term health and complex, chronic disease. In this way, Functional Medicine supports the unique expression of health and vitality for each individual.

How FM Changes The Way We Do Medicine?

Functional Medicine offers a powerful new operating system and clinical model for assessment, treatment, and prevention of chronic disease to replace the outdated and ineffective acute-care models carried forward from the 20th century.
Functional Medicine incorporates the latest in genetic science, systems biology, and standing of how environmental and lifestyle factors influence the emergence and progression of disease.
Functional Medicine enables physicians and other health professionals to practice proactive predictive, personalized medicine and empowers patients to take an active role in their own health.

In this occasion, I would love to share with you my mother's fight with Osteoporosis.
At the age of 40 and when her menopause (the discontinuation of menstruation known

by the word period) occurred associated with hormonal changes, her osteoporosis started to play a crucial role in her body and life.

Once, she got a small fracture in her leg and the Dr. confirmed, after examining her, that she was suffering from Osteoporosis. He, hereafter, subscribed her a few pills and advised her to increase her Calcium intake through milk and white cheese in addition to taking Calcium and Vitamin D supplements.

In spite of all the medications and vitamins, her Osteoporosis hasn't improved at all. On the contrary, it got worse, do you know why? In my opinion, it is because, during their hundreds of examinations, her Drs. never bothered to ask her in details about her health history, her life pattern, her food, her environmental changes, her habits and lifestyle. They only tackled the basic questions and directly moved to treat the symptoms.

They didn't examine thoroughly which medication might be good for her body since they've never treated her as an individual whose body might react differently from others. They didn't even try to foresee or look into the many factors that may affect her bones health in the long run. They didn't advise her with the right food which will nourish her body and her bones.

It's been 24 years now and mum is still suffering from Osteoporosis.And I strongly believe if she had been taken good care of by her Drs. at that time she wouldn't have reached this very advanced stage in Osteoporosis. In the past 2 years she had 6 operations in her hip and legs and wasn't able to walk. She broke 2 vertebrae of her vertebrate's spinal column and wore a cast for 3 months.

I've accompanied her several times to doctors' clinics and hospitals and not in one occasion did I hear them discuss with her the type of food she was eating. All they asked was whether she was taking her medications constantly or not.
Therefore, now I personally changed her food pattern and introduced her to healthy food that will nourish her bones and overall body. I eliminated the dairies and increased her calcium intake from fruits, vegetables and beans. I also bought her supplements that are food based.
Mum has a strong will and was always known to be an iron lady. Accordingly, I'm positive that the same way she cured herself in several occasions she will defeat her sickness this time and will feel great again. Every morning, she drinks vegetable smoothies and eats more raw nuts, fruits and vegetables and this has been going on for some time now. Furthermore, she stopped eating refined sugar. Her body is recovering again even though it is doing so in a slow manner.
Two years back, when she was in her worst health condition, and was barely able to walk, I challenged her. I told her if you start walking in the next 2 months I will cancel my summer vacation with my friends and will take you to Armenia, your mother country. My mom and I have never visited Armenia before.

She started working on herself and little by little we made it to Armenia. My brother Totix ("Tony" whom I like to call Totix) and his wife Roubzix ("Rouba" whom I've nicknamed Roubzix) joined us as well and we made mum's trip memorable. She walked a lot and we had to take lots of stops but her will was so strong that she intentionally lessened her pain. She enjoyed her country a lot and we all fell in love with Armenia's nature and its historical sites.

My recommendation to you my dear reader is first try to take care of your health in the natural way by leading a healthy and positive lifestyle and in case you needed medical help make sure to choose the right Dr. who will invest time in getting to know you as a person and not just treat your symptoms. I, for instance, never take pills for headaches or any other regular discomfort. I try to bear the pain as much as possible and trust my body to cure it and if the pain got worse only then do I ask for a Dr.'s advice.

Whenever you take a pill to reduce a certain pain, inflammation or kill bacteria, that pill breaks open in your stomach and gets absorbed. Your blood transports the chemicals in the pill to every part of your body. Antibiotic pills, for example, are medicines that treat infections caused by the approximately one hundred bacterial species that cause illness. However, the antibiotics don't often decipher the good bacteria form the bad ones. Hence, they destroy whatever bacteria they come across. That is why one pill may help you to decrease a specific pain or inflammation but it creates a new disease in the body. Therefore, listen to your body and try as much as you can to cure it in the right natural way.

❝ Eating right and leading a healthy positive lifestyle will keep pills & doctors away. ❞

Chapter Four

▪ **Healthy & Unhealthy F&B**

Health and weight management advisors recommend their patients to increase or decrease some kinds of foods to reach their targeted health goals. But unfortunately many people don't know the real benefits of the recommended F & B (food and beverages) and they consume unhealthy F & B regularly and abundantly.

Can you imagine the world 20 years from now? Can you imagine at what rate the percentage of diversified diseases, overweight, obesity and especially type 2 diabetes will sky rock? Can you imagine the health of our kids and new upcoming generations? Presently, the pre-diabetes and type 2 diabetes are attaining many kids and I assume new diseases will start to show up with the new kinds of food we are eating.

Let us therefore explore some of these food and beverages to understand better our healthy choices and keep food dangers away from our life and our loved ones' life.

1. Green Vegetables (GVs)

Types of GVs: Cabbage, Iceberg Lettuce, Red & Green Leaf, Romaine Lettuce, Broccoli, Mustard Green, Spinach, Swiss Chard, Collards, Turnip Greens, Kale, Chicory, Escarole, etc.

Why GVs?

They are essential to establish a healthy body and a strong immune system. GVs are highly oxygenated. They release the CO2 into the nature and absorb the O2. When you eat them, you will be receiving the clean O2 which strengthens the blood and cleans your respiratory system. Green Vegetables are for those reasons recommended to people with Asthma and respiratory allergies.

Now consider this, not many know that one of the essential minerals our body needs is the Alkaline, which is known to help our body neutralize the acidic conditions caused by the environment. Fortunately, GVs are high alkaline foods, and thus to consume a daily green vegetable diet or an oxygen-enriching diet is to help us balance and replenish the alkaline our body needs and continue to filter out pollutants. It is therefore crucial to keep in mind that green vegetables are necessary for people who are exposed to pollution.

What are GVs rich in?

GVs are rich in Calcium, Magnesium, Iron, Potassium, Phosphorus, Zinc and vitamins A, C, E, and K. They even contain small amounts of Omega-3 fatty acid. They are loaded with fiber, folic acid, chlorophyll and many other micronutrients and phytochemicals. GVs have very little carbohydrate in them and the carbs that are there are packed in layers of fiber, which make them very slow and easy to digest.

That is why, in general, greens have very little impact on blood glucose. Now if you don't have access to organic GVs, non-organic GVs are recommended because it is way better to eat the non-organic GVs than other kinds of processed and unhealthy junk foods.

I personally drink GVs smoothies in the morning. I mix 3 to 4 kinds of GVs with 1 or 2 kinds of fruits. Every day, I try whatever GVs and fruits I have available in the fridge and based on the taste I keep or change the ingredients. I as well mix many raw GVs in my salad and I include avocados in most of them as they provide me with the good fat that my body needs. For a change I steam carrots, sweet potatoes, eggplants and mix them with some lemon and virgin coconut or olive oil.

Benefits of GVs

Blood purification.
Cancer prevention.
Improved circulation.
Strengthening of Immune System.
Protecting cells from damage.
Regulating inflammation, and may help protect from inflammatory diseases including Arthritis.
Help protect bones from Osteoporosis.
Protecting eyes from age-related problems.
Improving Liver, Gail Bladder and Kidney function.
Clearing congestion, especially in Lungs by reducing the mucus.

How to Eat GVs?

In order not to get bored try a variety of methods. Start for example by mixing them in a salad and eat them raw. Fed up with that! Move to boiling them for less than a minute so that they don't lose their nutrients and get leached. You can also drink the water. Other alternatives to stay motivated are sautéing the vegetables in oil, sautéing them in water. Don't forget that if you overcook vegetable, they will lose their nutrients. For instance, overcooking spinach and kale will eliminate their nutrients. Finally try steaming which makes green more fibrous and tight and helps you feel fuller for a longer time.

2. Sweet Vegetables (SVs)

Types of SVs: Corn, carrots, onions, beets, winter squash, sweet potato , rutabagas, podded peas, turnips, parsnips, rutabagas,etc.

Why SVs?

Almost everyone craves sweets. Rather than depending on processed sugar, add naturally sweet foods to your daily diet to satisfy your sweet tooth. SVs soothe the internal organs of the body and energize the mind. And because many vegetables are root vegetables, they are energetically grounding, which helps balance out the "spaciness" people often feel after eating other kinds of sweet foods. Adding a sweet vegetable helps to crowd out unhealthy foods in the diet.

What are SVs rich in?

SVs are rich in vitamins (folate, vitamin B6, antioxidants like vitamin C, lutein, zeaxanthin, beta-carotene and beta-cryptoxanthin). Additionally, SVs are rich in minerals (potassium, magnesium, and zinc) and in fiber. Unlike poor-quality carbs such as white bread, regular pasta and other refined-grain products, SVs offer ample nutrition.

Benefits of SVs

SVs are a great addition to your diet when prepared in a healthy way. That said, starchy vegetables are higher in calories than non-starchy vegetables (like leafy greens, green beans, broccoli, cauliflower, peppers, cucumbers, carrots, mushrooms, and celery) so it's important to moderate your portions especially if you're trying to lose weight. Moreover, because of their high starch content, starchy vegetables raise blood-sugar levels more than non-starchy types. That is why individuals with diabetes need to be especially careful about limiting their intake of starchy sweet vegetables.

SVs are a good source of fiber. This can be rewarding since a high-fiber diet aids in weight loss and weight management because fiber fills you up quickly and staves off hunger. Moderate portions of starchy vegetables at meals (such as half a baked potato or half a cup of corn, peas, or winter squash) are a nutritious addition to any weight-loss plan. Finally eating a diet rich in fiber helps lower cholesterol and reduce the risk of heart diseases and strokes.

SVs promote as well some benefits to our health, which are listed below:

Reducing risks of cataracts and macular degeneration.
Keeping hair and bones healthy.
Contributing to the growth and repair of the tissues of the body.
Protecting skin against sun damage and keeping it healthy.
Decreasing the risk of developing inflammatory conditions, such as arthritis.
Reducing the risk of cardiovascular disease and slow age-related memory loss.
Warding off depression, migrane headaches, improving mood and combating PMS symptoms.

How To Eat SVs?

SVs can be cooked to your satisfaction. You can, for instance, empty the ingredients after cooking them into a large bowl,season them as desired and then eat. The leftover water makes a delicious sweet sauce and is a healing and soothing tonic to drink by itself. Other cooking methods include steaming, roasting, stir-frying. You can also try simmering and pureeing vegetables to create soup, or you can simply eat them raw, for example, grated in a salad. It is your court. Improvise.

3. Fruits

Fruits are packed with antioxidants, fiber, vitamins, minerals and other nutrients that can help you live longer, look younger, and even prevent you from diseases.

Types of Fruits

Blueberries,oranges,bananas,apples,kiwis,grapes,mango,limes,strawberries,plums, avocado, papayas, blackberries, cherries, cranberries, grapefruit,raspberries, watermelon, pineapple,etc. In general every fruit has benefits in a way or another and cures from some diseases.

Why Fruits?

Fresh fruits are nutritious foods that are a good source of vitamins, minerals, phytochemicals and fiber. Experts estimate that you should be eating five to nine portions of fruit or vegetables a day. However, if you are very much overweight or are insulin resistant, you should limit high sugar fruits (grapes, bananas, mangos, sweet cherries, apples, pineapples, pears and kiwi fruit) from your diet until your weight starts to normalize and your health improves. Note that some fruits (avocados, lemons, and limes) are very low in total sugar .Yet as I had previously mentioned, each body reacts differently, so all you need to do is just listen to your body and check your mood.

What are Fruits Rich in?

Fruits are high in Fiber, Vitamins A,C, B1, B2, B6, E, K, Folate (Folic Acid), etc.

Benefits of Fruits

Watermelon: Reduces ankle blood pressure.
Papaya: Protects against heart diseases and colon cancer.
Apple: Prevents from alzheimer, protect against parkinson.
Banana: Lowers risk of high blood pressure and strokes; prevents stomach ulcer.
Kiwi: Helps clean up toxins and protects DNA from damage.
Plums: Decrease anxiety.
Grapes: Fight heart disease.
Strawberry: Controls type 2 diabetes and staves off heart disease and inflammation.
Papaya: Improves digestion.
Cantaloupe: Boosts cell reproduction.
Blackcurrant: Prevents heart diseases; cancer; alzheimer and visual function.
Dragon Fruit: Lowers bad cholesterol (LDL) and raises good cholesterol (HDL).
Blackberries: Prevent cardiovascular diseases, cancers and osteoporosis.
Cherries: Reduce inflammation and lower triglyceride and cholesterol levels.
Grapes: Promote a healthy heart, slow the alzheimer's disease and break down stains and discolorations on teeth.
Pineapple: Good for digestion; helps break down food to reduce bloating.
Blueberries: Are good for better memory, boost metabolism, which can help keep you slim and energized.
Avocados: Lower LDL (bad cholesterol) levels while raising the amount of HDL (good cholesterol) in the body. Good for the heart health.
Cranberries: Prevent urinary-tract infections, fight ovarian cancer and slow the growth of some cancer cells.
Citrus Fruits (lemon): Counter the effects of sun damage and regulate oils and glands.

Eating Fruits

Fruits can be eaten raw as in smoothies, in a salad or in a meal. They can also be blended with a healthy cake or simply turned into ice cream by adding little corn flour to them. It's up to how you love their taste more and how you feel after eating them.

People wonder what time of the day is best to eat fruits. I say, all times are good as long as you are not feeling bloating, indigestion and any other malaises after consuming them.

Some say the best time to eat a bounty of fruit is either first thing in the morning on an empty stomach because the digestive process works very quickly, or as a mid-morning snack in between breakfast and lunch. Others say don't mix fruits with meals, because they will cause bloating. There's also this group of people who say it is preferably to eat fruits alone and not directly after a meal because the simple sugars contained in fruits need time to be completely absorbed by your body. Some advise not to have fruits before bed time as they increase your energy. Again I emphasize, there is no right or wrong.

Everything is related to your own system. You know your system better and you know if it can comfortably digest fruits during your meal or directly after it.
Personally, I like to have some fruits in the early morning or afternoon before my workout and I rarely have them at night before bed time and so far it has worked perfectly great for me.I eat dried fruits as snacks, for example, dates are my favorite. That's why my advice to you is to stop listening to what others say, eat what you like and listen **ONLY** to your body.

And the list goes on and on for different vegetables and fruits benefits, all you need to do is try few at a time and see how your body reacts to them. Some people, for example, have allergies on some fruits and vegetables. If you have allergy on a one specific kind of fruits or vegetables, this doesn't mean you have to stop eating all of them. Try the kind of fruits and vegetables that your body likes and eat them regularly. Be the mediator between your food and your body because only U can be the best auditor for your own health project development.

4. Nutrients

What is a Nutrient?

It is a substance that provides nourishment essential for the maintenance of life and for growth. Nutrients are the fuel of our body. If we don't fuel our system with the good nutrients our body will fail functioning properly. Take for instance the car, if we don't fuel our car with the correct gasoline, it will either stop or the engine will not run properly and sooner or later we will have to change it. However, in the case of our body, we cannot change it or buy another one as we only have One body. Therefore, we need to carefully preserve and protect it by being loyal to it.

The 6 types of Nutrients:

Food has more to it than simply satisfying your appetite as it undergoes a long process in your system after you consume it. The mouth is the only part of your body that tastes the bitterness, sourness, or sweetness.The stomach on the other hand digests the nutrients that will nourish your overall system. Note that each type of nutrient has a specific purpose and meets a specific need that your body has. The six nutrients are:

1. Water

Water is essential to life. Body composition varies according to gender and fitness level, because fatty tissue contains less water than lean tissue. The average adult male is about 60% water. The average adult woman is about 55% water because women naturally have more fatty tissue than men. Overweight men and women have more water, as a percent, than their leaner counterparts. The amount of water you need differs from person to person. It depends on various factors such as the type of activity you take part in, weather conditions, age, how much you weigh and how tall you are. Remember to drink extra water when you exercise, so your body doesn't dehydrate.

Let us look at the most important functions of water:

Cell Life: Water is a carrier distributing essential nutrients such as minerals, vitamins and glucose to cells.
Chemical and Metabolic Reactions: Water removes waste products including toxins that the organs' cells reject, and removes them through urines and faeces (also known as excrements).
Transporter of Nutrients: Water participates in the biochemical break-down of what we eat.
Body Temperature Regulation: Water has a large heat capacity which helps limit changes in body temperature in a warm or a cold environment.

Elimination of Water:

Water is an effective lubricant around joints. It also acts as a shock absorber for the eyes, the brain and the spinal cord.

2. Proteins

Proteins are like the brick and mortar of your body. They are the building blocks that provide the structure for the tissues of your body. Subsequently, We should eat good quality proteins like fish, chicken , nuts, seeds, beans and eggs.

An important protein composite, which recently the food industry is focusing a lot on, is Gluten. It is a glue kind mixture of proteins found in cereal grains especially in wheat grains. Hence, the food industry nowadays is promoting heavily gluten free labeled products because these proteins stick like glue and are not soluble in water causing in turn digestive disorders and illnesses such as celiac disease.

Many people feel discomforted after eating wheat, disregarding the fact that they might have intolerance to gluten. My advice to you is to check the signs your body is manifesting after eating any kind of food that is made of wheat and see how you will feel and decide accordingly whether it bothers your system or not. Your body might not react to gluten therfore you don't need to look for gluten free products.

The most accurate way to ensure that your food doesn't contain wheat is to read the labels.

Labels that contain monosodium glutamate (MSG), modified starches or malt usually contain wheat. Unless the label says otherwise, it is almost safe to assume that the food product contains wheat. Examples of food that contains wheat are abundant, for instance, flour, breads, baked goods (like cakes, cookies, pastries) pasta, pizza, breaded and battered food (fish sticks, fried chicken wings) cereals, canned soup, frozen or canned vegetables prepared in a sauce or cream, sauces, salad dressings, ground spices, instant drinks (coffee,instant tea, cocoa powder, malted and chocolate milk), desserts (like ice cream and puddings) condiments (like ketchup, mayonnaise), imitation and synthetic cheeses, beer, sweets(licorice, chocolate, candy with cereal extract),etc.

3. Fats

Fats are our storehouses of energy. When we have an excess of nutrients in our body, some of it is stored as fat. The primary purpose of fat is energy production. There are two main types of fats, saturated and unsaturated. Animal fats (meat, butter, lard) are usually saturated fats and may contribute to heart disease and cancer. Vegetable fats (olive oil, corn oil) are generally unsaturated fats and are less harmful.

Some fats have been found to be helpful in preventing some cancers and heart disease. These fats called omega-3 fatty acids are found in some fish, especially cold-water fish.

I personally get my necessary fat intake form fish, avocado, virgin coconut and olive oil, coconut butter, seeds, raw nuts, cashew and almond. These fats keep me healthy. Moreover they've helped me lose weight.

Many people believe that fat will make them fat "No fat will make you fat". It is the quality and quantity of fat you are eating that matters. Fat is essential to your system and you need to eat it in moderation.

Some people still believe that low fat food (cheese, chocolate, biscuits,etc), low fat dairies, skimmed milk, etc, are healthy. Alas!!! Do these people know that because low fat food doesn't taste nice, some food companies add sugar to make it tasty, Do they know that these low fat foods have less nutrients than full fat food and will make them eat more? What is more, I really don't know how people can consume this or can give the full sugary milk to their toddlers and babies thinking they are giving them good food.

For this my dear reader I entreat you to spread the word and help others with their food options. Shouldn't we all be aware of what we are eating?

4. Vitamins

The health benefits of vitamins include their ability to prevent and treat various diseases including heart problems, high cholesterol levels, eye disorders, and skin disorders. Most vitamins also facilitate many of the body's mechanisms and perform functions which are not perormed by any other nutrients.

Vitamins can be consumed in a variety of ways. Most common vitamins are acquired through the foods we eat, but your cuisine may be low in some natural vitamins. Therefore, the nutrition industry has made supplements available that can boost the vitamin content in your body. Personally, I consume my vitamins from the food I eat. And for those who have a job or a lifestyle that frequently causes them to miss meals, eat at different times, or eat the same food very often, I recommend food based vitamins.

Types of Vitamins: Vitamin A, Vitamin B1 to B17, Vitamin Bc-Bh-Bp-Bt-Bx-Bw,Vitamin C -D-E-F-G-H-I-J and Vitamin K. These Vitamins can easily be obtained by consuming different kinds of foods such as : Fruits, vegetables, meat,dairies, nuts, legumes, whole grains eggs, seafood,etc

5. Minerals

Minerals are compounds obtained from your diet and that combine in several ways to form the structures of your body. Different minerals have different benefits, so minerals cannot be termed as more beneficial or less beneficial than another. All minerals, even trace ones, are critical for the proper functioning of the body. Most of the minerals aid in body metabolism, water balance, and bone health, but they can participate in hundreds of other small ways to effectively boost health as well.

Types of Minerals: Calcium, Chloride, Chromium, Copper, Fluoride, Iodine, Iron, Magnesium, Phosphorus, Potassium, Selenium, Sodium, Molybdenum, Sulfer and Zinc. Minerals like vitamins can easily be obtained by consuming different kinds of foods such as: Fruits, vegetables,meat,dairies,nuts, legumes, whole grains eggs, seafood, etc. Many people barely give attention to their mineral intake. Now you know the importance of it. Eat food rich in minerals.

6. Carbohydrates

Carbohydrates are the primary source of energy for your body. Carbohydrates power every part of your body including your brain, heart, muscles and internal organs. They can be simple (table sugar, corn syrup) or complex (whole grain).

Our body's carbohydrates, fat and protein are the three main sources of calories known as macronutrients. After you eat carbohydrates, your body transforms them into glucose, a sugar your body uses as an energy source. If you learn how to choose your carbohydrates correctly, you will regulate your blood sugar, keep yourself in good and energetic mood, and thus avoid sugar binging and craving.

When you plan to eat in a healthy way, it is important to pay attention to sugar. Sugar is a major staple that provides carbohydrates. Natural and refined sugars are hidden everywhere. However, with a little extra knowledge, you can learn how to identify good sugars from bad ones. Accordingly, you can adapt your food intake. For this reason, you will be reading in the following paragraphs about the different types of sugar, their effect on your system and the possible ways to replace them.

Types of Sugar

a. Natural Sugar

Natural sugars are those carbohydrates that are an ordinary part of some food groups. For instance, fruits contain a natural single sugar called fructose. Milk and other dairy products contain both single and double sugars called galactose and lactose.

Other natural sugars include raw honey, maple syrup, agave nectar and molasses. I highly recommend the consumption of natural sugar because it is healthier for the body and it takes longer time to be burnt into energy than the refined sugar does. That is why the body feels full and energetic for a longer period of time say 3 to 4 hours. Subsequently, the body does not crave for more food or sugar after a short while of consuming them.

Therefore, the blood sugar level in the body will remain balanced and the body takes its normal time to breakdown the natural sugars and convert them to energy. As a result of this process no mood swings will be caused by our system.
There are some alternatives that you can use instead of the white sugar, such as: agave nectar, brown rice syrup, maple syrup, maple sugar, honey dates sugar, molasses, and vegetable glycerine.

b. Refined Sugar

Refined sugars are carbohydrates that supply calories with no nutritional benefit. Refined sugars are found in desserts, candy, alcohol, sodas, table sugar, etc. and are derived from processed plant materials including sugar cane and sugar beets. Refined sugars cause a rapid rise in blood sugar that could raise your risk of diabetes and other chronic problems. A large number of the foods we eat contain refined sugar, which could pose serious health problems.

Sugar is known as the "Entertainment Drug" as it is not less harmful than heroin. That is why you are on a sugar high when you eat candy and you feel good and energized for a short period of time until your body burns the sugar. After that your body feels down, your mood changes and you crave for more sugar and food. For this reason, after a lunch full of refined sugar people feel heavy, sluggish and tired and after a short while, say around 1 hour, they feel hungry again.

The processing of refined sugar strips away any fiber, vitamins, minerals and nutrients belonging to the plant and leaves a product that is almost 100 percent sucrose.

Increasingly more people are using the artificial sweeteners in their food thinking they are healthy and low in calories. But unfortunately, all sorts of refined sugars are bad for the health. They create an empty sugar buzz in the body, shaking the blood sugar level and the general function of the body for a short period of time.

After which the body will crave sugar again .This process will increase the blood sugar levels which in turn will increase the obesity and type 2 diabetes. If a person kept eating refined sugar soon many parts of his body, such as the eyes, feet, liver kidney, etc. will be affected and infected by diseases that are associated with diabetes.

The first thing I changed in my diet was to cut out milk, processed food, refined sugar, wheat, soda, chocolate, chips, artificial sweeteners and sweetened drinks. Furthermore, I used to drink lots of energy drinks during my daily workout and triathlons races. But, I stopped them all. My only best mate drink now is water. Even if I want to cycle for 6 hours and cross 150KM/day, I drink only water.

c. Lactose

Lactose is a sugar present in milk and other dairy foods. It is a disaccharide (also called Double Sugar, which is any substance that is composed of two molecules of simple sugars, monosaccharides, linked to each other) containing glucose and galactose units.

Some people have lactose intolerance and this means they have trouble digesting lactose. Lactose intolerance can be genetic and can happen to anyone at any age. Therefore, people should track their lactose intake. If they have an upset stomach or feel uncomfortable after consuming dairies, this might indicate their intolerance to lactose.

What does lactose intolerance mean? Well, people with lactose intolerance do not make enough lactase in their small intestine. Lactase is an enzyme that breaks lactose down into simpler sugars called glucose and galactose, which the body will absorb and turn into energy. Without Lactase, the body can't properly digest food that has lactose in it. This means that if you eat dairy foods, the lactose from these foods will pass directly into your intestine and this can lead to gas, cramps, a bloated feeling, and diarrhea.

Yes, a lot of people have lactose intolerance, but no one has to put up with feeling awful. If you have lactose intolerance, you can watch what you eat. I henceforth recommend 2 things. First, read labels carefully. Don't worry. Many processed foods are labelled lactose free, so indulge! Second, which I believe is very logical, convince yourself to decrease or cut out dairy products.

Finally, and if what has been said above caused you disappointment, I'd like you to consider this before consuming dairy products. Dr. Mark Hyman, MD, explained that milk causes acne, eczema, asthma ,skin problems, digestive disorders and the worst is that it can contribute to cancer and osteoporosis. Moreover, if you are careful about your weight, Dr. Hyman also asserts that even low fat milk can make you fat. No more disappointment if you like dairy products!!! Right!!! As for me, since I learned all this about dairies, I've stopped drinking and eating regular and low fat dairy products. As a result, the little acne I used to have on my face disappeared.

However, and once more, unless such types of food cause any disccomfort, don't deprive yourself from enjoying them. After all, my personal experience may differ from yours.

5. Low Glycemic Index

Glycemic Index (GI) is a measurement carried out on carbohydrate-containing foods and their impact on our blood sugar. GI is a relatively new way of analyzing foods. Previously, most meal plans designed to improve blood sugar by analyzing the total amount of carbohydrates (including sugars and starches) in the foods themselves.

GI goes beyond this approach by looking at the impact of foods on our actual blood sugar. In other words, instead of counting the total amount of carbohydrates in foods in their unconsumed state, GI measures the actual impact of these foods on our blood sugar. We rank our foods as being very low, low, medium, or high in their GI value. Therefore it is recommended while reading the labels to select food with low GI.
Low GI (0-55); Medium GI (56-69); High GI (70 or greater)

Did my recommendation so far help you to look deep into your food choices?Let us keep on exploring other healthy and unhealthy F & B and their effect on our bodies.

6. Aloe Vera

Aloe Vera is one of my favorite cactus plants that I would like to share its benefits with you. You may find this plant almost anywhere and its fresh juice is known to be one of the best juices you can have. You can mix it with your smoothies if they sometimes taste bitter.

Aloe Vera is rich in vitamins and minerals, such as vitamins A, C, E, folic acid, B1, B2, B3, B6 and B12. As for the minerals it contains Calcium, Magnesium, Zinc, Selenium, Sodium, Iron, Potassium, Copper and Manganese.
Aloe Vera is great for the cardiovascular health. It also boosts the immune system. It is anti microbial, anti bacterial, anti septic and anti fungal. I use it for my skin as it also increases skin elasticity, heals wounds and sunburns, lessens stretch marks and moisturizes the skin.It helps in digestion and promotes weight loss too.
I have an Aloe Vera plant at home and I make sure to eat a small amount of Aloe Vera gel every day.

7. Processed Food

What is Processed Food?

Processed food is commercially prepared food designed for ease of consumption. Subsequently the majority of people are consuming their calories and carbs from the processed food. Regrettably, they are doing so without having the real knowledge about the ingredients that create these foods. They are unaware that most of these foods are unhealthy and cause different diseases to our health. People think fat makes them put on weight, but in reality the junk processed food is the reason behind the weight gain and the type 2 diabetes.

Eliminating all processed foods from your diet may be quite difficult. However, you can significantly improve your health by eliminating the worst types of processed foods. Below is a clarification about healthy and unhealthy processed F & B.

I - Commonly Known Unhealthy Processed F & B

a. Hotdogs & Other Processed Meats

Hotdogs have been a staple of the American diet for decades. The National Hotdog and Sausage Council reports that Americans eat about twenty-billion hotdogs a year. They also report that ninety-five percent of all American homes serve hotdogs. Of course, lunch meats like bologna also have similar ingredient to hotdogs.

The vast majority of hotdogs and other highly processed meats on the market contain loads of salt, MSG (monosodium glutamate), sodium nitrate and other preservatives, in addition to artificial flavors, cheap unhealthy fillers, and mechanically separated meat and poultry. Most people don't realize that mechanically separated meat has been so highly processed under extreme heat and pressure that whatever nutritional value it had at first is lost in the process.

For example, proteins become denatured under these extreme industrial conditions. If you have an absolute craving for a hotdog , look for nitrate free organic hotdogs with no preservations, artificial flavors or meat byproducts. I used to love hotdog sandwiches until once I read an article that indicates the harmful ingredients that the hotdog consists of and I stopped eating them.

b. Soda Pop

There is nothing nutritional about sodas. They are empty calories. Moreover, they contain substances that can hurt you. As if sugar wasn't bad enough, many sodas today use high fructose corn syrup (HFCS) as a sweetener and this is even worse than sugar. HFCS has been shown to be damaging to the liver as well as causing blood glucose spikes even worse than normal table sugar would. No wonder Soda pop is a primary contributor to the obesity problem in the United States.

Soda pop is also one of the most powerful acid producing substances we can ingest. As such, it causes our naturally alkaline body pH to become acidic. Cancer cells thrive in an acidic environment and can't survive in an alkaline environment. An acidic body is also much more susceptible to viral and bacterial attacks since it weakens the natural defenses of the body's immune system.

Unfortunately, Soda Pop is the favorite drink for many adults and kids. Some prefer to drink diet soda without knowing that diet sodas and regular sodas are equally harmful to our system.

According to Dr. Hyman, the diet soda slows your metabolism, makes you crave more carbs and sugar and makes you store more belt fat. Some parents add water to the soda to decrease its acidity, whereas others knowing that soda is harmful for their kids allow them to drink it only once a week as a treat. And OH!! What a harmful treat!!

Personally I used to drink regular soda and diet soda recurrently when I was a kid. Then I decreased its intake during my teenage years until I decided to eliminate it totally from my dictionary. I henceforth recommend you to eliminate its intake. Now if you find it hard I advise you to decrease its intake to one small can per week and to drink it alone without any food until your system feels ready to eliminate it totally from you body.

c. Chicken Nuggets

Like hotdogs, chicken nuggets are at the pinnacle of industrialized foods. Most chicken nuggets are deep fried, often in oil containing trans-fat. Trans-fat causes cell membrane deformities that contribute to the development of metabolic diseases such as type 2 diabetes. It is quite alarming how obesity and diabetes are increasing tremendously among kids all over the world. In fact, more kids are found getting sick very regularly because of the food they are eating and paradoxically many parents wonder why their kids are feeling uncomfortable or have low immunity and are getting sick more often. I can't even recall when the last time that I had chicken nuggets was.

d. Store-Bought Cookies, Cake, Muffins & Crackers

Cookies, cake, muffins, and crackers have all been lumped into a single category because the health issues associated with them are similar. Beyond the obvious high levels of sugar and salt, most of these products also contain trans-fat. Trans-fat is added in small quantities because it is much cheaper than healthy fats and this makes it more profitable.

Moreover, trans-fat is also added to prolong shelf life and to improve the texture and flavor of the aliments. In fact, there are whole "food science" labs devoted to figuring out how to use trans-fats and other industrial foods to achieve the perfect texture in these types of products. Unfortunately many people consider these kinds of foods as the best sweets to fill their system with, without knowing their real effect on their bodies and how they shake the blood sugar in their system.

To know if a product actually contains trans-fat, you need to look at the ingredient list and look for the words "hydrogenated" or "partially hydrogenated". If these words appear, then the product contains trans-fat. That is why it is very important to learn how to read food labels. I used to eat lots of these sweets until I became best friends with my body and I started to be cautious about the food that I consume. Now I don't even get close to such food.

e. Many Popular Breakfast Cereals

Do you want to know why so many breakfast cereals are "fortified" with vitamins and minerals? Simple. The reason is because otherwise they would be so devoid of nutrition, no one would want to buy them. Fortified means the vitamins are artificially added during the processing of the food.

For example, these fortified cereals often add a form of vitamin D that is not easily digested by the human body.

Most breakfast cereals are also loaded with sugar or worse high fructose corn syrup. If they contain corn, as many do, then you can bet it is genetically modified (GMO) corn because this type of corn is much cheaper and this increases their profit. GMO corn has been shown to cause tumors in rodents in a recent study conducted in Europe. For this reason, I prefer to have boiled eggs, raw nuts, green vegetable smoothies and fruits than these unhealthy cereals for breakfast.

f. Nutrient Bars

The marketing of a few of the nutrient bars are remarkably deceptive. They are usually marketed as an exceptionally healthy food when in fact they are just the opposite. This means people tend to eat more of them thinking they are actually eating a super convenient, tasty, or healthy food when they really are not. Parents also tend to feel good about giving nutrient bars to their kids but they really aren't any healthier than a candy bar. People need to wake up and start to take a deep look at the food they are feeding their bodies and their kids' bodies with.

Regardless of what you see on the front of the packaging or hear in the commercials, few of the nutrient bars contain high fructose corn syrup. Even if they say they are made with honey or maple syrup, read the ingredient label. Some will put a tiny bit of honey or maple syrup for flavor but most of the sweetness is still derived from high fructose corn syrup. They are also sometimes loaded with fat including trans-fat, and lots of sodium too. Some Athletes or frequent exercisers highly trust these bars for their nutrient needs.

I, for example, spent almost 1 month eating 2 nutritional bars every day until I felt over frail and very tired before and after my exercise. I thought I could replace my meals with these bars, but I was very   mistaken and was about to cause serious damage to my body. Being an athlete, I learnt to never consider such nutrition bars a healthy option for me and I never ate these bars again.

After examining these food options, I would like to share with you a moving account. When I recently visited few of my friends who have kids and I told them about my new Nutrition and Lifestyle consultation passion, they felt motivated to undergo a lot of changes. They threw whatever candies, chocolate, cereal, nutrition bars and canned juices they have in their fridge and started to introduce the fresh fruits and vegetables options to their kids as healthy treats.

I just loved seeing and hearing how their kids started to love shopping for these treats and requesting them regularly instead of the unhealthy junk. This is to say everything is possible: **"When there is a will, there is a way"**.

c. Pre-Made Condiments & Salad Dressings

Some condiments and salad dressings contain high fructose corn syrup. Knowing that this is a really cheap way, food manufacturers can add them in bulk to their products and improve these products' flavors with very little cost. Condiments and salad dressings also contain transfats.

Another factor that makes them so unhealthy is that we tend to disregard what's in condiments when we apply them to our food. Even a healthy fresh vegetable salad can quickly turn into an unhealthy meal if an unhealthy dressing is added.

One way to eat healthier is simply to make your own condiments and salad dressings. This way you can control the ingredients. That is why, when I want to have food or salad in any restaurant, I choose my own healthy ingredients and dressings. I also ask the chef to make them for me, even if that means paying a little extra money, but at least I am positive I am eating right.

In conclusion, one of the healthiest steps you can take to improve your health is eliminating, or at least significantly reducing, the processed foods you eat. It is also important for you to carefully read the food label when shopping and not just depend on what it says on the front of the package.

II- Commonly Known Healthy Processed Foods

a. Canned Beans

Beans are an inexpensive source of protein and heart-healthy soluble fiber. Grab the low sodium canned version or rinse the beans in a colander under running water to remove 50 percent of the sodium per serving, according to the Academy of Nutrition and Diabetics. Sometimes, when I am in a hurry and don't have time for a long cooking process, I use these canned beans but I make sure to read labels well and choose the good ingredients.

b. Frozen Vegetables and Fruits

This is one of the best kept nutrition secrets. A recent study supports the current thinking that frozen vegetables and fruits are a nutrition bargain as they are as nutritious as fresh vegetables and fruits. Since frozen veggies and fruits are picked at their peak and immediately frozen to preserve their taste and nutrition, you can count on them for a serving of good nutrition right out of your freezer. Read the label to make sure you buy the varieties without the high fat sauces and high sodium seasonings added to the vegetables.

When you are running out of time, just take a frozen bag out of the fridge and cook it or do a smoothie with it. In fact, I sometimes use frozen vegetables and fruits in my smoothies although I prefer them to be fresh. But nothing halts the preparation of my green smoothie.

8. Alcohol

Why high intake of alcohol is not good for the body?

A glass of alcohol stays in the body for about 2 hours after being consumed. This period of time can vary depending on the person's weight, gender, and other factors such as age, fitness level, digestive system and general health.

When a person drinks alcohol, the concentration of alcohol in the blood builds up to a peak, then goes down. At first, alcohol often makes people feel relaxed and happy. Later, it can make them feel sleepy or confused. Note also that the small intestine and the stomach absorb most of the alcohol after drinking it. A small amount leaves the body through breathing and urinating.

If you drink lots of alcohol, you should try to decrease the intake of its consumption. Why? Simply and plainly because it causes lots of heart diseases. Moreover, kidney, liver, pancreas, and immune system problems are associated with the high consumption of alcohol. On top of that all, alcohol can be a party spoiler especially when many people drink alcohol until they get over tipsy, drunk or even until they vomit. This will not only spoil their outing but also annoy their surroundings.

Luckily for me, I haven't been allowed to drink alcohol due to my Judo training ever since I was a kid. That is why, I grew up not having the urge to drink it, and since then I have always enjoyed my time dancing and singing without surprisingly gulping down any kind of alcohol, and my friends of course have always wondered how I can enjoy my night and be so cheerful without any bit of alcohol in my system. As a matter of fact, I do very occasionally drink wine, and one glass can serve me the whole night.

9. Caffeine

What is Caffeine?

Caffeine is a bitter, white, crystalline, xanthine, alkaloid and stimulant drug. Caffeine is found in varying quantities in the seeds, leaves, and fruits of some plants, where it acts as a natural pesticide that paralyzes and kills certain insects feeding on the plants, as well as enhancing the reward memory of pollinators. It is most commonly consumed by humans in infusions extracted from the seed of the coffee plant and the leaves of the tea bush. Caffeine acts as a stimulant of the central nervous system.

Psychological Effects

The US National Institutes of Health states that too much caffeine can make you restless, anxious, and irritable. It may also keep you from sleeping well and may cause headaches, abnormal heart rhythms, or other problems. If you stop using caffeine, you could get withdrawal symptoms (listed below). Some people are more sensitive to the effects of caffeine than others. They should henceforth limit their consumption of caffeine; so should pregnant and nursing women do too because caffeine can have direct displeasing effects on their blood pressure, heart rate and babies' sleep patterns.

All kinds of caffeine are in one way or another harmful to our system if consumed abundantly, because they impair the absorption of calcium from the body.

Caffeine Withdrawal Symptoms

Withdrawal symptoms including headaches, irritability, inability to concentrate, drowsiness, insomnia, and pain in the stomach, upper body, and joints may appear within 12 to 24 hours after discontinuation of caffeine intake. These symptoms reach their peak at roughly 48 hours, and usually last from 2 to 9 days.

Coffee Dependence

Many People are coffee crazy! Coffee for breakfast, coffee for mid-morning break, coffee at lunch and finally afternoon pick me up coffee!

How many people we know cannot start their day without a cup of coffee or cannot even leave the lunch table without having their cup of coffee. More than that, if they decide to meet their friends, they also invite them for a cup of coffee. Yes!!! It is fine to consume a limited amount of tea and coffee, but not to the extent of addiction. Black coffee, for instance, may have some benefits if it is consumed as one cup per day and not after meals.

People who drink lots of coffee are harming their adrenals without realizing the long term bad effect of it on their system. How? Observe this. The well-known but poorly understood hormone adrenaline is produced by the adrenal glands from the amino acids phenylalanine and tyrosine.

When you eat protein-rich foods that contain amino acids, your body naturally produces these hormones and other brain chemicals that make you feel active and motivated and ready to get to work. If you take the coffee shortcut to get your quick fix of hormones you're exhausting your adrenals, the very organs you need to help you produce more hormones.

Like sugar, caffeine is a stimulant of the neurotransmitter serotonin which is a hormone in our brain that controls our sleep, mood and appetite. When our body depends too heavily on materials such as caffeine to control serotonin production and energy, the whole procedure impacts the body's natural ability to regulate healthy serotonin production. This is the reason for the highs and lows you may experience after a coffee.

On top of this, coffee tricks you into thinking that you're not hungry and hunger is our body's way of telling us that we need nutrients. My point is if we consume a drug (caffeine) that interferes with our hunger mechanism, we are depriving our body of the stimulus it needs to function naturally.

When we continue to top up on coffee further, we delay and deprive our body of nutrients, and the cycle continues in one big vicious circle. That is why those who consume lots of coffee during the day, feel full and with no appetite and unintentionally deprive their bodies from the nutrients and very soon they will get sick.

Some people will have sleeping disorders by only consuming one cup of coffee in the morning, but unfortunately they don't relate it to the coffee and they go wondering about what they have eaten or drunk before entering to bed without realizing that maybe the coffee they had had is the reason behind their disturbed sleep.

Therefore, if you are a person with sleeping problems, try to check whether coffee is the reason. How? Try to eliminate it for one week and check your sleeping patterns. You may feel sick and have headaches for a few days because your system is detoxing the caffeine, so bear with your body and continue checking your sleeping patterns afterwards. Coffee might be the reason behind your never ending interrupted sleep, you never know!

Finally, all kinds of coffee are not recommended in large quantities to people with osteoporosis because coffee impairs the absorption of calcium from the body.

10. Tobaccos

Though tobacco doesn't fall under the category of F&B, I thought it necessary to tackle it since it has become a crucial element of people daily dieting habits.

Smoking is extremely bad for health. That is why, all tobacco companies are constrained to list its cancer danger on all their packs, but still unlimited number of people smoke and do it regularly.

I have never tried smoking a cigarette so I don't know what or how people feel when they smoke. But one thing I guarantee is that if you are a person with a strong will and you usually achieve your set of goals in life, when you set your mind, quitting a cigarette will sound like a piece of cake for you.

For this particular reason I would like to share a personal experience about quitting cigarettes. My mum used to be a heavy smoker for almost 43 years, smoking 3 packs per day.

When I resigned from my job, I started planning for a detox trip to Thailand but mum was against this trip due to some political instability in Thailand at that time. I told you earlier, mum loves politics and she follows the world news more than the US president. So she started nagging, in an attempt to convince me to cancel my trip. I accepted on one condition which is: she has to stop smoking. Surprisingly, the next day I woke up, there was no smell of cigarettes in the living room. And when I kissed her the usual morning kiss, she smiled and said "Cancel your trip to Thailand Now". I was dumbfound but understood the message.

I laughed and said, you won't fool me with this. I am sure you will cheat, but she swore not to. Knowing my mum's strong will, I believed her and since then, in one forceful decision my mum has stopped smoking for good. I've started to share her story with almost every smoker I know, and I've kept on telling everyone that if a 64-year-old heavy smoker lady quit smoking in one minute, you guys can do better. Hopefully this experience will teach my smoking readers, **the power of will.**

I hope the above listed information is helpful and will enhance your food knowledge and make you select healthy choices. Many people who know me, like friends, relatives and colleagues remember me and smile while eating junk food and they either call me or just say to each other, can you imagine how Vicky will ironically praise us now if she was around. I am not a pain in the neck when it comes to food and drinks, but I appreciate people who really love and respect their bodies.

Before moving to the next chapter, I want you to challenge yourself for 14 days. I would love you to try my "Sweet 14 without Sweets".Try to cut out all refined sugar from your diet and see how your body reacts, how your mood becomes and how active you will be.

I tried it myself for 14 days and here I am with no sugar for almost a year. How many of us have set their minds on starting a diet on Monday, and then many Mondays came and went by and the diet was left behind. For instance, a person I know came up to her husband with the decision of starting a serious diet on Monday. He excitedly told her "so you are starting today?", and fast came the reply "no, I meant next Monday". Surprised he asked "why are you going to wait for next Monday to start?" She replied " I'm having a few friends' gatherings this week. Plus, my parents are coming over the weekend and I can't not eat with them."

The morale is simple:

" Don't postpone!!!
Start your makeover
today!!! "

Chapter Five

■ Make Healthy Cooking & Eating Your Hobby

Now that you've become an expert of food and beverages, it is time to hit the market and start picking those healthy treats for your friends, family and you. It's time to check your kitchen utensils and culinary items and last but not least learn how to enjoy healthy eating.

I know it is very difficult to see the billions of tempting food packages on the shelves with their mouth-watering low fat labels, seductive pictures and catchy promotions and not buy them. But I am sure by now you are well aware what their successful marketing campaigns hide.Seems difficult to implement? Don't worry! I'll be sharing with you some of my shopping, culinary as well as eating secrets. Buckle up and enjoy the ride.

Food Shopping

After learning and understanding about the healthy and unhealthy food and what types of food are suitable for me and compatible with my digestive system, I started to love going food shopping. I enjoyed going alone, or with my friends, and with whoever asked me to accompany him. I also advised them how to shop healthily. Fruits and vegetable sections in the local markets and supermarkets became my favorite spot. I never again approached the low fat chocolate and chips, unhealthy processed food, meat and dairies aisles.

Things have changed quite enormously for me. Now you could see a big smile on my face while choosing my vegetables and fruits because I know they will keep me healthy and energized. Picking them has become like a treat to me. It's like I had a special positive connection with them.

Shopping List

I make sure my weekly food shopping list covers around 70% for my fruits and vegetables and 30% for the remaining food such as fresh fish, organic chicken, raw nuts (almonds, pecans, pistachios, walnuts, cashew,etc), hummus, organic beans, olive oil, coconut oil and other healthy options.

Food Investment

I always advise people to invest in their food the same way they invest in buying the best brands to wear. I believe the internal textile of our body is more precious than our external textile. So invest the best you can in your food because its effect is everlasting, whereas clothes, accessories and cars' effect lasts until a new fad hits the runway.

After-all, making a commitment to healthy eating is a great start towards a healthier life. Beyond eating more fruits, vegetables, beans, and good fats there is the question of food safety, nutrition, and sustainability.

How foods are grown or raised can impact both our health and the environment. This brings up the question: What is the difference between organic foods, conventionally grown foods and GMOs?

1. Organic Food

To start, organic foods are free of synthetic chemicals, are grown in nutrient rich soil and are not treated with pesticides or chemical fertilizers.

To continue, organically raised farm animals are free of antibiotics and added hormones. These animals are not allowed to have their genes modified. They are raised in healthier environments with so much care and respect and are organically fed, and often eat a wider range of nutrients than animals in factory farms. Moreover, organically raised animals are not bred from a test tube.

Furthermore, organic produce contains more vitamins, minerals, enzymes and other micronutrients than intensively farmed produce.
According to a research published in the journal of Agricultural and Food Chemistry, organic fruits and veggies have 50% to 60% higher levels of cancer fighting antioxidants than non-organic fruits and veggies.
Hence,it is preferable to buy organic produce whenever possible, but if the budget is an issue, don't let that put you off. You will still benefit from non-organic produce but choose the good options.

In all cases, consider this when you feel reluctant about your shopping: though organic food is more expensive, the extra money you pay may save you hundreds if not thousands of dollars in future doctors' or pharmacies' bills.

I, for example, try most of the time to eat organic products. Nevertheless, if for a reason or another I couldn't get a specific product I read the labels well and choose the best provided.

2. Conventional Foods

Conventional foods are currently the standard produce and are grown using synthetic chemicals such as fertilizers and pesticides. These chemicals then get absorbed into the soil and cannot be removed.

The purpose for conventional farming is to mass-produce. In fact, conventional farming allows for out of season growing, and creates a longer shelf life. This type of farming uses monoculture. This means crops are often planted over and over in the same place which leads to more insect infestation and diseases, and this also depletes the soil of nutrients. Farmers are then compelled to use more fertilizers to kill insects or prevent the spread of diseases.

This endless cycle often leads to massive topsoil erosion. Hence, it is believed and somehow widely spread that conventionally grown foods are tasteless due to all the chemical treating.

3. Genetically Modified Organisms (GMO)

Genetically Modified Organisms or GMO's are the new thing spreading in grocery stores. These foods have been genetically altered. Scientist now can essentially cut and paste different genes into produce. The purpose of which is to make this produce resistant to pest, grow quicker, taste different, etc.

Obviously, if you could grow fruit without pesticides and still have it turn out perfect, then it would be a wonderful thing. However, there are issues with GMO's. First of all there is the allergy issue. Since we can cut a gene from one food and paste it into another, then it can possibly transfer the allergy causing part to a new food. Thus if someone is not allergic to a normal apple, they could be allergic to a GMO apple because it might have a gene from a food they are allergic to.

So in one word, we need to carefully check what we are eating. I, for example, love to buy from local farmers. In Lebanon we have a lot of farms where only organic food is produced and I can feel the farmers' positive energy in all the produce they reap and sell with cheaper costs than the stores which sell organic food. If I am unable to find such farmers or buy their produce, I buy the organic food from real organic shops where pure organic produce is sold. Even though the price is higher in the latter shops, my health is more important than anything else.

Recently some organic shops are promoting their products to be organic, whereas they are not. So be careful while choosing.

Sadly there are still a lot of people who eat poorly and feed their kids with bad choices. Long time back cancer disease was an unfamiliar word, now it is infecting every house, every gender, and every age in multi different ugly ways.

Shopping for Canned Food

When I want to buy canned foods I read labels well. I try to avoid lactose, High GI, refined sugar, and unnecessary ingredients with difficult names to pronounce.
I take my time to read the labels and understand each ingredient. I do this only once for the products which are new to me until I become familiar with them. This means the next time I see them, they go into my trolley if they had been compatible with my digestive system.

Reading Labels While Shopping

Though it can be time-consuming at first, food shopping must mean label shopping. HOW? Easy. Keep this in mind. Healthy to me means to choose non-labeled real foods or foods with 5 or less familiar ingredients.

Reading labels and knowing what you are eating can become so much fun. It is normal not to know the names of all the ingredients. For that, try looking up the unfamiliar ingredients on the net. I, for instance, often do that when I buy a new product and I don't know one of its ingredients. I Google them on the spot, and accordingly decide whether to buy the product or not. I personally don't eat one single ingredient without checking its details. For this reason, I learnt how to read labels and now I enjoy exploring them.

I now smirk when I check a product with multi-ingredients and complicated names, and I wonder how I used to buy things without even checking what they are made of. I also recall the many times my poor body digested these foods silently and complained to me through the ailments it exhibited while unfortunately and unintentionally I used to ignore the signs.

Expiry Dates & Shopping

I always check the expiry date of any food I am buying or eating as some food become very contaminated after their expiry date. Hence, I prefer the non-labeled food such as vegetables and fruits because they contain no added ingredients and you decide their expiry date by personally checking their freshness.

A friend of mine once told me she consumed products 1 or 2 days after they've expired. She was totally unaware of the dangers of her behavior and was like "it's only a day or 2". This simple answer was enough for me to lose my temper and start lecturing her about the poisonous products she was consuming. Moreover, her act brought to my mind the thousands of people doing that. And yet, we are panic-stricken, astounded, enraged, and sickened when we hear someone has caught a deadly disease or when a dear sibling, son or daughter had a virus and more when this close person died.

Luckily for my friend, after sounding the alarm, I managed to touch her sense of logic, and when we met again, I learned from her that she'd stopped eating expired food. And that every time she threw them, she remembered my furious face and how I'd reacted and she smiled.

As happy as I was for her I wished I could raise more awareness to the many people I come across while shopping. I wish I could alert them. I also wish I could convince you so that each time you go shopping and watch what you or others are putting in the trolleys, you remember me and smile. Actually, I do want you to remember me with a smile, not only by watching others' trolleys, but as well while reading labels and filling your trolley with healthy choices.

Just rest assured even though I sooo want it, I won't be around watching you.
To finish, I want to recount to you something I have seen and have been smitten by. I recently saw one couple I know through a common friend shopping in the same supermarket where I happened to be. They are known to be successful executives in the corporate world. Now, when I looked at their shopping cart, I felt so bad seeing all kinds of unhealthy food choices. It struck me how such highly educated people with lots of money are feeding their bodies with terrible food and raising their kids on very bad and unhealthy food. Their shopping cart was full of unhealthy processed foods, canned foods, biscuits, chips, sweetened juices and many refined sugars. At that moment I wished I had known them more so I could shared few tips with them.

Your Beautiful Kitchen - Your Pharmacy

As I mentioned to you earlier, the kitchen had always been a grey area for me until suddenly it became one of my favorite zones where I improvise to prepare food for my friends, my family and me. The kitchen to me now is my pharmacy, it's the place from where I get the good medicine, namely the healthy food, for my body. After my weekly shopping I bring my bags to the kitchen, and nothing enters the fridge and the kitchen cupboard without being cleaned well. I surely don't want to fill my kitchen with bacteria. Hence, check below few steps that can help you keep your kitchen clean and ready for healthy cooking.

1. Your Fresh Fridge

You can tell the eating lifestyle of people by checking their fridge and finding out what their food choices are based on. I, for example, clean my fridge on a weekly basis knowing that it is a hotbed of lots of bacteria that could harm my family and me. Thus, I make sure I always clean my fridge properly then put my clean healthy food back in it.

Unfortunately some people don't even clean their fridge for a month, year or more. And yet, they clean their houses on a daily basis, specially the floor. They probably feel lazy to clean their fridge as it might take time and some extra effort; disregarding the risks they're up to. Disregarding the fact that even if the floor is clean, bacteria can still be present around their house and kitchen. Subsequently, their system recognizes them during digestion and this can affect the health of their bodies and loved ones, which I'm sure no one is in favor of. Therefore kill the germs before they harm you and harm your family. To do that, here are some tips that can come in handy.

Store the only healthy washed, clean and well-packed stuff in your fridge.
Use more glass jars for storing than plastic boxes.
If you are a mum or a dad, approach your kids in a fun way to make them assist you in the cleaning process. Hold them responsible of handling some cleaning tasks depending on their age. For instance, ask them to wash or dry some fruits or vegetables. You may treat them afterwards with some fresh smoothies; they will love it for sure.

(The purpose behind this activity is not to facilitate the cleaning process on you. The purpose is to teach your kids how to love healthy foods and to teach them how to take care of themselves. This small initiative will create good habits in your kids and they will remember you every time when they clean their own fridge and kitchens in the future. By being good healthy models to our kids, we forge good and healthy generations.)

Use special solutions to wash each and every piece of your fruits and vegetables. (I use lemon, vinegar or salt to wash them). Choose whatever product you want, but the most important step is to clean the market food you bring home. Clean the canned products and everything you buy from the market, you don't want the market germs to surf in your kitchen cabinet and between your kitchen stuff.

(Your kitchen and fridge are your healthy image, so keep them fresh, shining and clean.)

Pack the leafy vegetables well in a cloth or a clean glass jar, whichever you want but remove them from the polluted market bags.
Replace the market bags with your clean bags.
Wipe things that are not washable with naturally sterilized products. (I use lemon and baking soda).

(I like to use natural cleaning and skin care products and I always search for new combinations.)

Finally, to wash all the foods that you bought, might be time-consuming and sometimes you might not be in the mood for it. You could simply be tired or you have to run for a meeting or a gathering. So you decide not wash the items, and shove them as they are in the fridge.

I do understand all that. I myself get engaged many times in activities and feel the same and it's normal to encounter all these obstacles. But…But…But…when you prioritize your body and your family's health and understand the hazards of not doing this, and when you imagine the bacteria flying in your fridge, then I am confident that you will invest more time in accomplishing your weekly cleaning of food shopping.

It will take you a few times to incorporate this habit into your kitchen routine. Don't worry soon it'll be a joy especially once you start to save time during cooking knowing everything is ready to be cooked. What a delight! Especially if you are a working person and you're always on a tight schedule.

In the past my fridge used to contain few cans of diet soda, few sweetened juices, my favorite chocolates and biscuits, few cans of tuna, low fat cheese and yogurt, 2 or 3 pieces of cucumber and some fruits. Whoever used to open my clean fridge in the past, used to directly know that I don't cook and I live on partially healthy food. But now, whoever checks my clean, fresh and organized fridge, they can directly tell that I am a 100% healthy freak and that I cook healthy foods. I have all my items nicely and neatly washed and packed and you can easily serve yourself without doubting about the cleanliness of the food.

2. Kitchen Equipments

They are very essential as they assist us in making our food process healthy. Therefore, we need to keep them highly maintained, sterilized and in a very good condition.
I visited many kitchens and I saw very old tools which are still being used for cooking. People don't realize the importance of these tools and how they react with our foods specially while cooking. Hence, and in order not to put your health at stake try the following tips:

Always try to search for and buy the best quality and read the manufacturer's details well to know how to use them.
Avoid using metal or hard plastic utensils on cookware. These utensils can scratch surfaces and cause pots and pans to wear out faster.
Do not use a scratched pan because it will release toxic chemicals to your food which may affect your system and cause discomfort to your body or may create a kind of disease.
Do not heat dry empty pans, they may cause toxic particles to become airborne and embedded into your lungs through the food you are eating.
Always have oil or liquid in a pan before heating or inserting any food in it.

3. Fun Cooking

I love this part. I love to have fun and inject love in whatever I am doing. Who could have ever imagined that one day I will take up cooking?

I used to laugh when I read in some resumes that cooking is their hobby, and I used to say to myself "Look at this hobby. Hello people!!! Go get a life!". But look at me now, yes, it is happening, and yes I am enjoying cooking a lot and it's becoming my hobby.

Of course at times it happens that I am not in the cooking mood, but I have to prepare a meal. I, therefore, pause for a second, breath, and jump to the kitchen with full of energy and I start cooking.
How can I do this? I can enjoy anything I do by just tuning the atmosphere a bit. I do the same while exercising. I'd love to share with you below a list of things I do and that would hopefully pump up your cooking mood.

Enjoy listening to your favorite music.
Breath calmly and deeply.
Don't cook if you are not in a good mood, you might have a stomach ache afterwards or feel discomforted because you will be putting negative energy in the food.
Remember you are cooking to a loved one. It could be yourself, your parents, friends, wife, children, etc.so put your love and positive energy into your food.
Involve your friends, parents and family in your cooking.
If you are a mum, you can plan a weekly activity with your kids and husband.
Ask them to prepare you a nice meal or smoothies once a week. They can search on the net and be creative in preparing something yummy. *(I, for example, like to improvise and try new recipes that I learn from a cooking program on TV or from a cook book.)*
Introduce new and fun approaches to your kids to love vegetables and fruits. For example, invite their friends over for a fruit or vegetable party and let them make their own salad and smoothies and the best mix wins a prize.
Plan a family day cooking and let everyone enjoy their share in cooking.
Let the kids watch their dad cook, then take photos of him, and finally post them on their Facebook page for their friends and themselves to enjoy.
When the weather is good, try to prepare the salad or the smoothies with your family on the balcony and ask the kids to run to the kitchen and assist you with getting the ingredients. *(I like to prepare my salad on the balcony and enjoy the nice breeze.)*
Avoid using unnatural cooking materials, such as the microwave.
Food made at home and food made at restaurants are not the same.

At home our grandmas, mums, or us prepare the food with all the love and positive energy we could give. On top of that, we always guarantee to offer the best food and best taste.

On the other hand, in the restaurant some of the chefs and their team are under stress. They have hundreds of dishes to prepare. They might be in bad mood and thus working with high negative energy which believe me, in a way or another, will penetrate your dish and cause you discomfort.

Considering all that, try to reduce eating outside your own beautiful clean kitchen. It is good for your health and your pocket as well.

I, for instance, manage to eat 80% home cooked food and 20% restaurant light salads.

It is worth mentioning that every time I go to a restaurant I ask to meet the chef and have a nice quick conversation with him before ordering my food because I want to give him an incentive to put his positive energy while preparing my food. At least I am positive that now he will try his best to make it healthy and delicious to win my positive feedback. As a matter of fact, I had chefs who came back to my table to ask me about the dish and listen to my comments.

However, since meeting a chef is not always possible in busy restaurants, I always try to design my own ingredients with the waiters and as I mentioned earlier I like to have my sauce placed at the side with the ingredients I want. I don't mind paying a bit more to get healthy stuff in my salad or dish.

In the end, like many of you I always appreciate the good dishes in the restaurants but I also love to thank the chef who's prepared them for me. "A smiley and kind thank you" plays a big role in comforting and making others feel great. Try then to use them very often for almost all the good things happening around you.

Eating & Digestion

The digestive system is a series of hollow organs joined in a long, twisting tube from the mouth to the anus. Inside this tube is a lining called the mucosa. In the mouth, stomach, and small intestine, the mucosa contains tiny glands that produce juices to help digest food.

So digestion is about chemicals reacting between the food we eat or the juice we drink, and the enzymes our system produces. Moreover, our digestive system needs different enzymes (maltose & maltase) to digest carbs and amino acid to digest proteins, therefore when we eat rice and chicken together, we will be tiring our digestive system in producing multi enzymes to digest our food which on a long term might cause digestive problems and creates diseases.

So eat slowly my friend, no one and nothing is more important than the food now entering your system. Feel the process, close your eyes and imagine how bites are being processed in your system. It is fun, believe me. We can't do this all the time, but we need to give it our best.

Here are some tips to good eating.

Cook once and eat twice. How? Eat the food over two days for lunch or dinner. You can savor it at home or at work.
Avoid overly cooking the food, because overcooking will kill the nutrients in your food. Eat more raw food. Enjoy blending and juicing especially in the summer months.
Try to have a glass of the smoothies you've prepared at home as a meal. I choose smoothies for breakfast. It is very easy and fun to prepare. Blend some of the veggies and fruits you have in the fridge and drink. What is the difference between juicing and smoothies someone may ask? Well, the difference is that while juicing

you only extract the juice from the fruit or vegetable leaving the fibre in the pulp collector at the back of the juicer machine. Therefore the body doesn't have to break down and digest any fiber. The nutrients in this case are assimilated in a matter of minutes rather than hours. When preparing smoothies on the other hand, the whole food is blended into a thick drink using all of the fruit except for the skin and seed. Consequently, smoothies are great as the fibre from the fruit provides sustenance, fills you up and gets your bowels moving. Many people don't like specific fruits or vegetables, but they can bear them in smoothies or juice.

There are very practical blenders in the market that don't need lots of washing and high maintenance. If you don't have one, get one **NOW** and kick off your juicing and smoothies treats.

Alter your eating habits to more simple food. Simplify your cooking and flavorings to get a simplified taste and a simplified way of living.

Keep your salad sauce light and simple. My favorite salad sauce includes lemon, vinegar, olive or coconut oil.

Try to avoid adding flavors in the food you're preparing at times. Place a tray of a variety of flavoring and condiments on the dining table and let each one add his own favorite flavor and check their feedback. If they like it, you can do it more often. It will decrease your cooking time.

Have small bites and enjoy every bite you take.

Don't keep your fork in your hand, relax, chew slowly, and afterwards pick your fork and have another yummy bite. Don't rush and give time for your stomach to digest peacefully.

Chew, chew, chew and chew your food. 50% of our digestion process occurs in the mouth. Eat slowly, concentrate on your small bites and remember your stomach is like a blender if you fill it quickly and to the top, it will take you ages to digest. When your food gets in contact with saliva it becomes wet, making it easier for foods (notably dry ones) to pass easier through the esophagus. **"It ain't what you eat but how you chew it".-- Delbert McClinton**

Eating slowly and chewing are equally important because saliva contains enzymes that contribute to the chemical process of digestion.

Carbohydrate digestion begins with salivary alpha-amylase secreted by glands positioned near the mouth.

Fat digestion also occurs in the mouth with the secretion of the enzyme lingual lipase by glands located at the root of the tongue. So enjoy chewing well your fatty food.

Incomplete digestion may lead to bacterial overgrowth. So smash your food well before swallowing them.

Before starting your meal, close your eyes, put your hands on the top of your plate, smile and be grateful for what you are eating. Remember many don't have food to eat.

I personally prefer to eat carbs and protein separately. For example I eat vegetables with carbs (salad with beans and gluten free pasta or brown rice) and vegetables with protein (salad with fish, chicken, egg, etc). I fill my plate with 70% vegetables and 30% with other group of foods. I like to fill my plate with a colorful variety of vegetables to brighten it.

Preferable to drink water and juices before or after 30 minutes from any meal and not during. Mixing liquid with food might cause bloating or digestion issues. But again, if you feel comfortable drinking liquid with food, do it. The most important thing is for you to feel great. But now you know that if you felt any discomfort, this could be from the liquid with food. Test, test, and keep on testing your food with your body signs. It is your body and you know best what is good for you.

There are lots of healthy foods that are good for you. Don't necessarily go for the ones that have been recommended to you by others and you can't stand.
Avoid heavy buffet brunches, lunches and dinners. Your body doesn't need all kinds of these food groups combined at a time. You will make your system suffer instead of nourishing it with good, healthy, and balanced food.

I personally don't like to go to buffet restaurants, and if I go, I try to eat simple and not mix many food groups together. People think that at the weekend they are free to eat anything. Even more, some other people choose one day per week to eat anything they want freely. I don't really understand this concept, why do we have to wait for the weekend or a vacation to eat whatever we want. Eat everyday whatever you want but choose healthy options that suit your body. If you become loyal to your body, you won't wait for any special occasion to eat right. Every day is a special free day for you.
Fuel your body with the real food because you only got one body to accompany you until the day you leave this life. Invest in it well.

Finally enjoy eating your food everywhere. Enjoy it in all the different ways, for example, alone, with friends, with colleagues, with family, outdoor, indoor, surrounded with candles, by moonlight, or in fresh air. Do anything that makes you feel happy but the most important thing is to focus on the food flow and enjoy how your body is being nourished from inside.

"Be the engineer of your own body & health. At the end, as they say... U are what U eat."

Chapter Six

Add Energy To Your Years

Do you want to reach your 70 or 80 years in a healthy and energetic way? Start investing in your health now. It is never too late to start. Just stand in front of the mirror and take a deep look at your figure and imagine yourself after 20 or 30 years. Do you think you will be a healthy and active mum, dad , grandpa , grandma or a fit single bachelor? If you know so then good luck to you. If you feel you need maintenance, start your self renovation project now and enjoy reaching your 70 or 80 healthily and happily.

I have come across many 70-year-old people cycling, running and swimming. I was astounded to see them release a burst of energy even when they were only walking. Contrarily, I have 20, 30 and 40-year-old friends who can barely move and who suffer from numerous health problems. A few of them take medicaments on a regular basis,why? It is the outcome of their lifestyle **CHOICES**.

Sports – My Passion

As I had previously shared with you, I started Ballet dancing and then Judo at the age of 5 and since then I have been in love with Judo and all kinds of sports.

I used to train Judo at Bouddha Sports City ,where i also used to manage kid's summer and winter camps. Bouddha is known to be the number one sports club in Lebanon owned by Mr. Francois Saade who is the President of the Lebanese Judo Federation and who played an effective role in building healthy and sporty generations for more than 30 years. Personally i was inspired by Mr. Saade and for the past 20 years Bouddha was my second home where i spent long hours with my sports colleagues training kids to practice all kind of sports and helping them make their marks in the sport world.

My passion to sports grew day by day. I was my school's basketball team captain and I also participated in all kinds of sports. I practiced skiing, horse-back riding, gymnastic, ice skating and won many prizes in inter scholar track and field tournaments such as in shut pull, javelin, high jump, long jump, short distance run, 5k and 10 k run. I used to participate and win in mostly all of the tournaments. In short I was always the dynamic girl who grew up having adrenaline rush in my system all the time.

Sports have remained my passion till date. I never say no, for a sports invitation. I actually plan my outings to be on sports courts so we can either go running, swimming, cycling or play tennis and squash. And my friends joke with me by checking whether my date passed my fitness test or not.

Going back to my eating habits, at a young age I used to exercise and eat without knowing the importance of both. I did them as part of my daily routine. I am sure my parents as well as most of the parents don't have the accurate knowledge about food and nutrition therefore sometimes I was fed with the correct meals before my sports tournaments and sometimes with wrong meals which made me feel weak, sick and tired during and after the games.

I travelled to different countries and participated in many International Judo tournaments. I have encountered a lot of funny and exigent experiences, but I want to share this particular one that was a bit challenging.

I had to participate in an International Judo championship in Canada, where I had to lose 7 kg in 3 weeks. It was on very short notice but I had to do it anyways. At that time, neither my coaches nor my parents had good nutrition awarness and thus the choice of meals was basicaly left to me. I mainly depended on the thought that I am strong, and I said to myself "no worries V you can do this". Henceforth, I didn't eat anything and drank weight loss unhealthy shakes. Of course, I reached Canada tired and energyless. I had still one kg to lose before my next day game. I ran,used the sauna facility and didn't drink any water or eat any food the whole night so that I could reach the suitable desired weight.

The next day in the morning at 6am, I got on the scale and as you can guess I passed the measurement test and had to get ready for my game at 2pm. You can imagine how I was feeling and how I looked. Yes, I was exhausted but still excited for the game. I had 6 hours to eat before my game, but I barely ate some fruits and drank water because my system was rejecting any other food due to the stress I had undergone.

When I started the game, I was unable to play well, actually I felt over dizzy and about to faint most of the time. I had a double vision, and could barely concentrate on my opponent. It's like I was having a blackout.In spite of all that, I survived the whole game without surrendering, but without a doubt, I lost. Yes, I lost, but I learnt one thing: never to stress my system like this again. Unquestionably since then, if I had to lose or put on weight, I started to plan better eating habits.
This game taught me to convey better messages to my Judo students. I used to share it with them followed by good nutritional tips.

I kept doing Judo during my teenage years and I had consulted lots of sports nutrition specialists. All used to give me different advice following their different school's beliefs, so sometimes their advice worked and sometimes it did not.

When I started to travel for work, I wasn't able to continue my Judo practice but I never stopped sports. I shifted my energy to other kinds of sports such as Swimming, Cycling, Running, Squash, Tennis, Ping Pong, etc.

Being a sports freak, and always prioritizing early morning exercise especially at week-ends, I had to sleep and wake up early. So most of the time I missed my friends' loud parties and yet, this didn't keep me from enjoying quality time doing sports with the group of friends that are as sporty as I am.

I have suffered from a chronic lower back pain due to an accident while I was playing Judo 15 years back. A 95 kg male colleague fell on my back while training and smashed my L1,L2 and S1 vertebras. This pain can put me in bed for a few days, while being unable to move, but that never stopped me from doing sports. I relax for a few days then kick off again a mild exercise routine including lots of Swimming, Pilates and Yoga.

Throughout my life, I have never stopped exercising for more than one week, until very recently I had to stop exercising for 3 months. I was so much on low energy that I felt like dying.

Recently, I had a minor hand surgery due to a cycling injury. Consequently, I was in a recovery stage relaxing my hand and undergoing physiotherapy sessions for almost 2 to 3 months. This was the longest period in my whole life during which I had to stop exercising and I learnt a lot about the human body.

I learnt that if you don't move your muscles, you will become very lazy, no matter how active and athletic you are. What is more, your muscles will hurt you and make you think it is better to stop exercising .Contrarily to this assumption,when this happens, your body is telling you that you need to move your muscles as they are becoming very stiff.

I, myself, experienced this for the 3 months when I stopped exercising. In fact, my whole body was aching. I was feeling down, lazy and not in the mood to even go for a long walk. I used to go hiking and swimming on Sundays and afterwards feel tired for the whole week. This really startled me because I could usually exercise for 3 hours in a row per day without feeling tired. But at that time, I was not even thinking about sports. I was enjoying my studies on the expense of my frail muscles. I never imagined I will have this feeling and attitude towards exercising. Then I realized how the human body can get used to a certain boring monotone that will make him lazy and out of energy.

I started recalling all the alibis that I used to hear from my clients and friends about exercising. For instance, they used to repeat: "I don't feel like exercising, it is boring for me; I am tired; I don't have time; I don't know where to start; I don't know what is the suitableexercise for me; I don't like running or cycling, I don't have a nearby good gym and I don't like to drive; I come late from work; etc.". It was only then that

I understood their situation clearly. I was having the same attitude towards sports throughout the 3 months I spent recovering form my hand injury.

Fortunately for me, I regained my balanced exercise pattern after my recovery period. I went back to my active exercise routine, and I learnt new ways to motivate people to exercise.

Bottom line, if we keep our body in its comfort zone for a long period, it will be more challenging to refresh it back or to put it in the right healthy track again. But this does not mean we should give up on our body and on ourselves. Remember nothing is impossible. It's all about the mindset. Believe me, I've lived it and I know it works.
Now try the following when you are suffering from any injury, so you don't restrain from exercising entirely.

If you have an injured hand or any upper body injury, workout your lower body. You can, for instance, go running and walking, or even do lower body weight lifting exercises in the gym or at home.
If you have an injured leg or any lower body injury, workout your upper body. Swim or do upper body weight lifting exercises in the gym or at home.
Yes, you might always feel tired, lazy, not in the mood, etc, but what you need to do is fight your thoughts, motivate your senses and throw yourself into an active sports pattern again. Always think that the human body needs 21 days to change an activity into a routine or a habit.

Think of your own body and regain the good relationship with it.

How To Begin or Restart Exercising?

Wawooo,I just love this topic.It stimulates my energy and I feel this particular question is on most of the inactive people's minds.
Same as cooking, to enjoy exercise you need to know the anatomy of your body well, how it works and which sports are enjoyable for you. You cannot just stick to your old school and university exercise habits. You need to experiment new sports and see what your body likes. There are lots of people who started cycling, diving, skiing, swimming, etc. at the age of 40, because only then were they introduced to these sports. Of course, they wish they had tried it earlier.
I will share with you some beneficial information and tips which I am positive when followed, will help you kick off a healthy sporty lifestyle.

1. Set Fitness Goals and Work on Achieving Them

Firstly, keep in mind that all kinds of sports are fun. This means all you need is to check which ones your body calls for. Some people, for example, like adventure sports. Others however like Yoga and there are those who are keen on outdoor activities, or fitness classes, and so on. I, for instance, love sports that give high adrenaline rush. I love skydiving, mountain biking, cycling, skiing, snow-boarding, etc.

Secondly, all sports have risks, some low, some medium and some high.

So choose a kind of sport that fits your physical ability. If you have any severe injury or health problem, it is better to refer to your practitioner. Although consultations might not work most of the time, but still it's better to check with your Dr. which kind of exercise you should enroll in. For example, my Dr. wanted me to seize running and cycling because of my back problem, but I never stopped either one. I know my body well and I know its limits as well. When I feel pain, I take it easy.

Thirdly, whatever sports you choose, please make sure you do a small research about its rules and risks in order to avoid any injuries and accidents. That is why, I recommend each person to have a personal trainer or a coach to assist him at the beginning of his sports kick off.

Then, remember that to reach your specific fitness needs, you need to set fitness goals. Decide what you want. Like for example: How many kilograms do you want to lose or gain? Do you need to tone or firm your body? Do you want to tighten or strengthen specific areas in your body? Do you need to reshape? Do you finally want to start Mediation, Yoga or Pilates? Do you wish to participate in a 5k or 10k run? Do you want to enroll in a mini or full marathon? Are you interested in learning new sports or in competing in a swimming tournament? Do you want to join a group in touring the city on bike? Do you just want to walk, listen to your favorite music and relax? Keep in mind that the purpose of exercise is not only to enhance your figure, it is also to help boost your mood, and improve your stamina and sex life. Moreover, exercise helps to keep diseases away and helps you to think positively.

Finally, undertake some sports that you like but never really tried before and check your enthusiasm towards them. If you got motivated start immediately. This is what I actually did. I'll recount my happy discovery of my love of cycling.

It all went like this. I saw a very cute 60-year-old Austrian couple putting their bikes in the car and going cycling. Uffff, they inspired me big time. I do indoor cycling (spinning) and I used to have a little small bike when I was a kid, but never really cycled outdoor for ages.

Subsequently, I approached them and introduced myself. I asked them some questions about their cycling practice. "Ohhh yeah!!!" I got more motivated when I heard about their programs, what they do, where they cycle, and how many hours per day/week. I was literally amazed by them. They cycle 6 to 8 hours at weekends, they cycle 150 k per day, they run and swim. They are Triathletes. (Triathletes, means they participate in Triathlon races).

The lady saw the energy and excitement in my eyes and told me "Since you sound very interested, why don't you join us tomorrow?" I had a big grin on my face, delighted at her offer and excitedly said "thank you, soooo sweet of youuuu, I'd love to, but I don't have a bike". She said, "no worries honey, we have an extra one that I can lend you". I wish you could feel my happiness at that time. I was literally jumping in my place like a 4-year-old girl who's just got her birthday present. I was like "Reallyyyy, so I can ride with you tomorrow???" she confirmed "well yes, only if you want." My mind was repeating those phrases breathlessly: "Only if I want to???, Are you kidding me???"

I hugged and kissed this beautiful stranger lady who now became my lovely 60-year-old active friend Theresa. And then I've cycled weekly with her husband and her for some time. I bought my first red sexy mountain bike, then another attractive red road bike. I also joined a few other cycling groups. Later, I motivated one of my active 40-year-old friends Roberto Khoury, who started to join me in cycling and almost all the activities. Afterwards, I created my own cycling team called "Whats-Up Team" to motivate new cyclers and especially people above 35 and up to 70 to start cycling. I used to enjoy people kicking off their exercise routine by joining my cycling team.

Later, I joined Theresa and her husband, who took my breath away with their energy, for one of their triathlon races after which I completed my first triathlon and motivated Roberto to join me as well and since then our triathlon journey has continued.

The message behind all this is that you too can do the same. You can try cycling, hiking, running, swimming, etc. All you have to do is to throw your body in the sports healthy courts and let it choose nice sports for you. Choosing an active sports partner can motivate you too.

I have a colleague who started motorbiking at the age of 50. Motorbiking had always been his passion but he only had the opportunity to try it at 50. He loved this activity and bought his first motor bike and started to have long weekend drives with a group of bikers. He enjoyed every minute of it, and it boosted his lifestyle. No matter how old you are it is never too late to exercise and regain your energy. I just love it when I see during my triathlon or marathon races people in their 50s, 60s and 70s running, cycling, swimming and having fun. Some people are 30 years old, but walking around with a stiff body of a 60-year-old person. Others I know are the exact opposite, 60-year-old with the body of a 30-year-old.

If you are already a person who exercises regularly always try to vary your sports activities in order to exercise other specific muscles in your body. When I started cycling, I started to feel the move of many new muscles, which I used not to feel before. That is because each sport is designed to move different muscles.

2. Choosing An Appropriate Venue For Your Exercise

Based on your fitness goals, choose a place that is suitable for your practice and that fits your busy daily schedule. I personally prefer outdoor activities unless it's too hot or too late at night. In this case, I switch to indoor facilities.

I love the beautiful nature in Lebanon. I love to hike, run, cycle, and do outdoor activities all year round there. There is one particular person in my lovely family who inspires me big time. He's my 68-year-old auntie's husband Joseph Atallah (Tonton Zuzu, as I like to call him). Do you know why he's inspired me? Well, in addition to being a lovely and caring person, he is one of the most active people I have ever met in my life. He used to accompany me while I was hiking, and he hikes better than the 30-year-old guys in our hiking group. It is worth mentioning that he never hiked before in his life. When he was young, he used to go swimming and running but never tried hiking. What is quite interesting is that he started this activity at the age of 68. How amazing and inspiring is that? Moreover, he is so much in shape that he can go past other hikers easily.

Does Tonton take any medication or energy pills, you may ask? NO, he is an active and healthy person who's managed to eat healthy and exercise daily throughout his life. He can walk 3 to 4 hours on the treadmill every day. He can walk outdoor for 4 to 6 hours. Yes, he inspires me and he's inspired most of my friends when they saw his hiking pictures. They went like "wawoooo…he managed to hike all that in 6 hours?" And my friends got motivated and started to join our hiking group. I love you Tontonaaa and I wish you more positive and healthy energy to your life.

What I like as well in Lebanon, is when in February, March and April, I go skiing in the morning and then directly hit the beach for a swim. It's an amazing feeling which to my knowledge you may not experience in any other part of the world.

a. Fitness Clubs

Many people include exercise in their monthly and New Year resolutions. Everyone plans to start doing new sports, buying a new gym membership or sports attire at the beginning of summer season or at the beginning of every New Year. Little however keep up to this resolution.

Neila Rey says: **"I already know what giving up feels like. I want to see what happens if I don't."** And thus in order for you to see what happens if you don't give up, try the following:

Choose a gym close to your work or home.
Make sure the management and the staff are customer oriented. Check what ways they implement to keep you tuned and motivated. Do they do follow up calls in case you were away for a while?
Check staff and management promptness and friendliness. Check customer care system in case you needed any assistance.
Inspect the general atmosphere of the facility and level of customers; do you enjoy such a crowd?
I always recommend subscribing for 1 or 3 months membership to try the services before enrolling in one full year membership.
Check their hygiene standards and whether they are equipped with advanced machines.
Check their programs and if they do regular fitness assessments to track your fitness progression.
Check their consistency as service providers. Do they have consistence fitness classes and one on one personal training sessions?
Check if their prices are in line with the market.
Check if their operating hours meet your schedule.

After examining all these areas, it will be easier and more comfortable for you to decide whether this gym is the right one for you or not. And after you subscribe for one trial month you will have an adequate feedback and decide whether to enroll and benefit from their yearly offers or not.

b. Outdoor Facilities

Where can you get fresh air better than from outdoor areas. The favorite place where I enjoy the energetic breeze and beautiful natural scenery is the outdoor facilities or open space arenas. Even in hot countries I used to enjoy the fresh air outside.

Choose a safe place for any sports you are willing to undertake. If you want to exercise after your work and you think the nearby area is a bit unsafe at night, invite a friend, a neighbor or motivate your partner to join you. You will have a chit chat with a nice walk or jog.

When I wanted to buy my own new house in Lebanon, my first concern was to find a nice area where I can practice my running. I got lucky and found a good location surrounded by trees and nice natural views.

3. Sports Attire

After you choose the kind of sports you want to practice, get the proper outfit and accessories to avoid any injuries. If you don't know which outfits are the most suitable, simply ask the sports shopkeeper for assistance. Furthermore, make sure your body is sweating in a healthy way to avoid any allergies. Check your sports shoes. It is recommended to change them every 6 months especially the running ones.

4. Water Bottle

One of the important things you should always have with you during exercise is a special sports water bottle so you don't get dehydrated or simply to satiate your thirst.

Water is truly a vital source for the human body. You need to drink more water per day if you are exercising. Imagine that you can survive a month or so without food but only 5-7 days without water.

Water is at the center of life. For that, even if you don't exercise, it is recommended to drink 2 to 3 liters per day. One way to facilitate that is to put an alarm every 30 minutes to remind you to drink water.

At work, I tell my team not to offer me any coffee instead to fill my big cup of glass with water every time they see it empty. So I manage to drink around 3 liters per day during my office hours. During my exercise, I drink additional 2 to 3 liters.

It is recommended to drink the daily required water amount throughout the day before 7 or 8 pm. If you drink water late at night, your body may react differently and your sleep may be interrupted causing you to visit the washroom more often. And yet, needless to remind you that you should listen to your body as you may be from those people who are not affected by too much water consumption.

I have met few people in my life who never drink water but drink fresh juices in return to compensate for the water and stay hydrated. Again, we come back to the bio individuality theory. Listen to your body.

5. Heart Rate Monitor

Many people don't know the benefits of monitoring their heart rate during exercise. It is one of the best ways to keep yourself on track and avoid unexpected injuries. Your heart rate is a convenient, reliable, personal indicator of the intensity of your exercise. It's good to know the intensity of your exercise so you can vary it depending on your fitness level and the goals you want to achieve by exercising. Heart rate monitoring benefits you in the following areas:

Assists you in controlling your intensity and gets you to avoid being hard on yourself. Provides feedback on your improvements and motivates you to progress better in your trainings.
Tracks your improvement.
There are professional athletic watches that can measure your blood pressure, heart rate, track your speed and distance, offer data transfer, navigation and GPS, count your food calories and your daily steps,etc.These watches are my toys.

6. Meet Your Muscles

Unfortunately, throughout my fitness journey, I have met lots of athletes and fitness lovers, who surprisingly have no clue about their muscles. And it makes me feel bad when a person doesn't know what lies within, what makes him move and live. I surely don't expect everyone to be an expert or a doctor, or to memorize the anatomy of the body. But at least, if you want to move your body properly, learn about its basic parts so you can exercise safely and effectively.
Therefore, it is very crucial to learn briefly about the muscles of your body and be aware of how your system is functioning.

a. Our muscle tissue has the ability to relax and contract and so brings about movement and mechanical work in various parts of the body.
b. Muscle is the tissue of the body which primarily functions as a source of power, and can be divided into three main groups according to their structure:

i. Smooth Muscle Tissue: Smooth muscle contracts involuntarily, without conscious intervention and is found in the internal organs, such as the digestive system, and it can stretch and maintain tension.
ii. Cardiac (Heart) Muscle Tissue: Cardiac muscle contracts involuntarily and is located in the heart and both stretches and contracts.
iii. Skeletal Muscle Tissue: Striated or skeletal muscle only contracts voluntarily, upon influence of the central nervous system. Skeletal muscles, considered the major group of muscles, are attached to the bones by bundles of collagen fibers known as tendons that are held together by connective tissue. Here comes our role to keep this group of muscles refreshed, alive and active by exercising.

Almost 99% of the mass of the human body is made up of six elements: Oxygen, carbon, hydrogen, nitrogen, calcium, and phosphorus. Only about 1% is composed of another five elements: Potassium, sulfur, sodium, chlorine, and magnesium. All are necessary to life. Therefore we need to supply our system with sufficient nutrients, enough sleep and recovery period to keep them highly maintained.

7. Personal Trainer

I highly recommend people to hire personal trainers and coaches, especially if they are new to a workout pattern or to a new kind of sports. I, as well advise personal trainers for moderate exercisers who need to learn new techniques and be motivated.

Moreover, I suggest that everyone schedules meetings with the personal trainers before enrolling in their programs. Let them offer you a trial assessment session to see if your energy meets their energy. Check what certification they hold because in many gyms they hire unqualified people to save money.

Pour on them all your questions and examine how knowledgeable they are, try to figure out their hygiene level as this can be a turn off especially if they have a bad sweat or a bad breath, which may annoy you during the session.

There are many benefits of hiring a personal trainer which can be summarized in the following points.

Customized one on one sessions may assist you to reach your goals faster and in a 90% effective way if the trainer was highly qualified and knowledgeable.
Most of the people need motivation, therefore hiring a personal trainer can fulfill your needs. They can push you hard to reach your optimum results.
They can share with you many tips you've never known about fitness and nutrition, although some of the personal trainers have basic nutrition knowledge.
With the supervision of a qualified fitness trainer, you can secure a 90% free injury training session.
They will inform you about all the machines in the gym, so you can use them safely whenever you feel you want to exercise alone.
They can be good companions who will share with you your chosen sports.
They will periodically analyze your body composition through fitness assessment tests, so you will know exactly your progression results which will motivate you even more to stick to the program.
Personal trainers and coaches are like any school teacher, if you like him/her you will love the subject. I, for instance, had encountered in my team some fitness trainers whose clients used to love them and stayed loyal to their programs for years. On the other hand, I had few clients that complained about other trainers who talk a lot during the sessions, share unnecessary jokes and sometimes interfere in the clients' personal life, which made the clients shift to another trainer.
Every sports has its own risk and rules which personal trainers and coaches share with their clients to avoid risks and injuries.

Even if you are tight with your budget to hire a personal trainer, I recommend you to book at the beginning of your exercise journey one or two personal training(PT) sessions to know the basics of the exercise you have chosen after which you can exercise alone.

Get motivated and stay tuned. I wish you all the luck in choosing your perfect fitness trainer.

8. Music

Download your favorite music on your phone or your iPod and make sure to have it while practicing any sport because as we all know music is an energy booster. It can fire you up or calm you down, both in a nice soothing way.

I have 3 different iPod cases, one for cycling, one for running and a waterproof one for swimming which I use while I am pampering my body in the waves. The waterproof iPod case allows me to swim for almost 2 hours without feeling tired. The rhythm of the music swims with my senses in the water and takes my breath away. If you have your iPod on while the gym music is playing, monitor the volume not to annoy others. It is very irritating when you have your loud iPod music and there is someone exercising next to you who wants to either enjoy the gym music or just focus on his training peacefully. Moreover, It is also irritating when you have to answer a call while you are exercising in the gym or when you are talking very loudly to a friend who is exercising next to you. Some people might get annoyed, so better watch out.

9. Breathing

And now after you managed to explore almost all the necessary requirements to kick off, to restart or to balance your fitness activities, it is time to know the importance of breathing in everything you do including exercising.

Breathing is special in several aspects: it is the only function you can perform consciously as well as unconsciously, and it can be a completely voluntary act or a completely involuntary act, as it is controlled by two sets of nerves, one belonging to the voluntary nervous system, the other to the Involuntary (autonomic) system. Breath is the bridge between these two systems. Unfortunately, the majority of people take breathing for granted, and do not know how to breathe.

Knowing how to perform simple breathing techniques can help lower the blood pressure, calm a racing heart, or help your digestive system without taking drugs. I manage to remind myself to breath slowly many times during the day and I feel just great.

Breathing has direct connections to emotional states and moods. Observe someone who is angry, afraid or otherwise upset, and you will see a person breathing rapidly, shallowly, noisily and irregularly. This explains why you cannot get upset if you breathe slowly, deeply, quietly and regularly. Of course you cannot always center yourself emotionally by an act of will, but you can use your voluntary nerves to make your breathing slow, deep, quiet and regular, and the rest will follow.

Breathing is the most important act, without breathing and oxygen there is no life. Yes, we can survive a month or so without food, or a few days without water but we can never survive few minutes without breathing. So breathing is the optimum characteristic of our health which we don't unfortunately focus on. It is therefore crucial to focus on our breathing throughout the day not only while exercising.

Breathing has unlimited benefits. Here are a few:

It detoxifies and releases tension.
It relaxes the mind/body and brings clarity.
It relieves emotional problems and pain.
It strengthens the immune system.
It increases the digestion and the assimilation of food.
It improves the nervous system.
It strengthens the lungs and the heart.
It assists in weight control, boosts energy levels and improves stamina.
It improves cellular regeneration.
It elevates moods.

Breathing is the one and only exercise that all livings mutually practice to stay alive. Therefore proper slow breathing during exercise or non-exercise time is essential for the general wellbeing.

Some Indian beliefs say if you breathe slowly, you will live longer. I always recommend meditation, because it teaches you the proper breathing that your body enjoys.

If you want to live long, breath like a Turtle, which is known to breath very slowly and live long.

Motivational Fitness Tips

1. To start , I recommend disconnecting from everyone for an hour or so and put your phone on silent mode while you are exercising.

2. Exercise minimum 3 times, one hour per week, then start to increase your exercise hours and days up 4 to 5 times/week, from 1 to 3 hours per day especially during the weekends.
Remember that when we exercise, our bodies release the hormone Endorphine, which boosts our minds positively and makes us happy. That is why most of the athletes or people who exercise regularly are always energetic and in high spirits. And when they refrain from exercising for a while they will be cheerless.

3. If you are new to the exercise pattern or have just recovered from an injury, start walking 3 times per week for 15 to 30 minutes. Check and write down how many meters you are walking in this timeframe. After a week increase your intensity and again check how many meters you are walking/jogging in 15 to 30 minutes. Keep it up like this and you will smile when you see the results are progressing successively. You will be motivated to throw yourself in the outdoor area or in the gym very frequent. Walking and jogging make your brain stronger and enables it to grow healthier.
After my rehabilitation, I tried to run 5k. And Oh!!!! It was like a burden, my body was weak and I was a bit down. Before I could run 10km quite easily. And the

fact that I couldn't pull this through kind of saddened me.But I talked to myself and decided to take it easy.(I love self-talk, it makes me realize what thoughts are surfing inside my mind and makes me more conscious .) For the first week I ran 1km and wrote down how much time it took me. I did it in 7 minutes at first and then slowly I went up to 6 minutes/km. I gradually tuned my knees and legs again and regained my score of running the 1km in less than 5 minutes.

4. Record your efforts every time and compare them to your last record.

5.Try to incorporate strength training in your exercising schedule. Strength training burns lots of calories and reshapes you well. Try exercises like using dumbbells, machines, your own body weight (by doing squats, push-ups, set-ups, etc). Many ladies don't like strength training as they fear to form bulky figures. However, and according to the Women's Heart Foundation, high levels of estrogen make it very difficult for women to become overly muscular. When women lift weights in moderation the changes to their muscles are generally related to tone, strength, and endurance rather than size. The resulting look is firm, feminine toning not bulky masculine muscles. It as well helps in preserving muscle mass, controls weights and reduces the risk of osteoporosis. Strength training helps preserve and enhance your muscle mass, regardless of your age.

6. If you are not familiar with the gym machines, let the available personal trainer in the gym advise you on how to use them to avoid unnecessary injuries.

7. Do not weight lift without having the correct knowledge of how to use and lift your muscles or the machines. You will harm your body.

8. To avoid injuries, always warm your muscles up at the beginning of the session and stretch at the end.

9. Your muscles need to recover after each effort and exercise. This is very essential.

10. To avoid any discomfort, don't exercise directly after your meal, allow 2 to 3 hours time for your body to digest the food properly.

11. If you like you can have a small piece of fruit 30 minutes before your exercise to stimulate your energy and prepare your body for the proper energy burning.

12. If you want to lose weight, I recommend not to eat 3 hours before exercising to allow your body to transfer the stored fat into energy. Still, this is up to how you feel and what signs your body shares with you. Listen to your body.

13. If you had a long day at work or did lots of movements during the day, it is recommended to shower before hitting the gym or starting your exercise. This will avoid the flow of any bad odors.

14. If you are a mum or dad, enroll your kids in sports activities and drag them away from the indoor electronic games/internet. Seed in them the love of sports.

Coach them how to live a healthy life starting from their early age. Trust me by being a good example, your kids will look up to you.

15. Organize sports activities with your kids during the weekend like hiking, running, cycling, swimming, tennis, wall climbing, kayaking, pedaling, etc.

16. Organize a sports day for all the kids and adults in the family, or invite all your friends to bring over their kids for some funny sports activities. Don't wait for any special occasion to get together, create the occasion and enjoy a healthy sporty day with your family.

17. Improvise active plans. Don't play the role of boring parents. Initiate tight bonds with your kids, grandkids, nieces, etc.

18. If you are single, prepare some funny sports activities to your nieces, neighbors' kids or friends' kids. It is a good idea to stay close to kids as to prepare yourself to becoming a parent one day.

19. Why not involve your kids, partner, or friends in preparing weekend activities in order not to feel bored. For instance divide tasks among you, one weekend you organize the activity and the other weekends them.

20. Buy a road or a mountain bike and enjoy outdoor activities with your family.

21. Keep the childhood spirit always alive in you. Growing young is the best way to enjoy an active happy life.

22. Find an active sports partner that you can count on to motivate you while you are feeling lazy.

23. Motivate your partner and organize some games for couples such as tennis, squash, ping pong, etc. Inject healthy activities in your daily life. Exercising will enrich your intimate gatherings and rejuvenate your physical performance.

24. Join your friends for aerobic and anaerobic activities, it is fun and a way to network and get motivated.

- Aerobic activities provide cardiovascular conditioning. Aerobic activities mean the activities where breathing controls the amount of oxygen that travels to the muscle and helps them burn fuel and move. These types of exercises use oxygen to burn fat and carbohydrates to produce energy. They are activities like fast walking, running, skiing, cycling and swimming. Aerobic exercise usually involves the whole body.

- Anaerobic activities promote strength conditioning. Athletes use anaerobic exercise to promote strength, speed and power. The bodybuilders use the anaerobic exercises to promote muscle mass. Anaerobic exercise needs more oxygen than your body can give. Anaerobic exercise involves a specific group of muscles and burns only carbohydrates, such as sprinting, high intensity interval training, power lifting, basketball, tennis, football and most athletic sports.

- We need to mix aerobic and anaerobic activities within our exercise routine.

25. I believe group activities are very motivating. Search on Facebook or within your community for road biking, mountain biking, hiking and swimming groups who will keep you tuned.

26. If you are a housewife and cannot join any gym, get some aerobic CDs , invite your neighbors' housewives and friends to enjoy a group class instead of a coffee chit chat.

27. If you are an employee or student, keep your sports attire in the car and move directly from work or university to the gym for some refreshing exercise. Many people go home after work or university to rest, or pick up some stuff, before hitting the gym, but they end up watching a movie and eating popcorn on the lazy couch.

28. If you think you are that very busy overloaded person and cannot manage 30 minutes per day for your body to go for a run or hit the gym, then the easiest way to do is to invest in a home treadmill or any cardio machine. In this way you have no reason to skip the 30-minute daily exercise. You can run on the treadmill while you are watching a movie or some fun talk shows. I know many friends who have treadmills at their houses which they used a few times then turned them into hangers or decorative item in the corner of the room because they are never used. My recommendation is to place the cardio machine in a very strategic location in the room, for instance, in front of the television. And rather than being a couch potato go ahead and jog on the treadmill. You can as well do like me and find yourself a nice movie to watch while putting yourself to work.

29. If you are a cycler and riding on the road, never have any type of music instrument on. You need to keep all your senses clear and stay concentrated on the road and cars to avoid any accident or injury. We are learning about lots of death cases where drivers are smashing the cyclers. Personally, I ride in the early mornings where few cars are on the road and I keep my eyes and ears wide open. We all want to enjoy our sports in a safe way.

30. If you are a diver, make sure you are well-equipped and have an experienced body (diving partner is called "a body") with you before any dive.

I'd like to benefit from mentioning diving to recount a horrific incident that happened to one of my best friends. I do hope this story will spread awareness and be an example that may save other people's lives. My 29 - year - old best friend's name is Joseph Bou Rached. He was my inspiring sports partner in Judo, diving and almost all the sports activities. We used to organize together skiing, ice-skating and cycling trips to our school students during weekends. I have learnt a lot from him.

Yozo (as we all like to call him) was a healthy and fit Judo champion who used to practice diving in his spare time. He wanted to immigrate to Canada, and so as a farewell trip, he and his friends organized a diving trip on Sunday 09-10-2004. They were 6 divers. Once in the depth of the sea, one diver panic and the 6 divers faced some challenges. Yoso assisted the 3 divers to reach the service then he went back to assist the other 2...and since then I've missed him and many also missed the 3 altogether, as we lost them to the sea.

He was supposed to travel to Canada, the next day, but destiny took him and 2 of his friends to a place where their beautiful and innocent souls are dwelling in peace. They found their bodies in a cave, where apparently they had been lost and struggled to find their way out. I miss you Yozo. Since then I stopped diving as I promised my parents not to. Yozo was a kindhearted, sweet, smart and professional person and the challenges he faced at the bottom of the ocean were buried with him.

He could have saved himself but he used his last breath to save his friends. He died a hero practicing his favorite sports. Bottom line: All kinds of sports can be risky and dangerous, but we need to be always cautious and well-equipped.

31. Last but not least, If I ever felt lazy to go to exercise, I do the self talk and it goes something like that "Excuse me you need to go to your exercise, your body needs to relax and get some fresh oxygen". This is enough to motivate me, make me smile and put me on exercise mode.

" Make exercising your daily routine & kick off your healthy lifestyle today... "

Chapter Seven

▪Self Care

The minute you invade the world, you invade it with a partner, your body, the body that breathes without any effort coming from you. This body will accompany you throughout your life and will die with you.

At your early life stages your body takes care of you and communicates freely and effortlessly with the surrounding environment to protect you because you are not yet ready to face the real life alone. Your body initiates a relationship with your parents or guardians who feed it, so it can develop properly. It communicates with your parents what you like and what you dislike. Haven't we all been at one time newborns or toddlers with frustrating eating patterns? Haven't our bodies refused to drink milk, or eat some kinds of vegetables and fruits, or even digest specific kinds of food, etc.? (ask your parents they sure have loads of those stories to tell you about).

At this early stage of life you are not aware of the events happening around you, you have no control over your breath, moves and food. You only show contentment when you are fed well, and annoyance when you aren't fed well. Your acts are summed up to 2 things mainly, smiles and cries. Your body assists you involuntarily to do that. Your system communicates with your surroundings, to explain to them what is happening to you.

You are only a receiver until you start to walk, talk, eat and drink voluntarily. Only then do you start to understand what is happening around you. You grow dependent of your guardians. You trust them because they were the ones who welcomed you first to this world, and you feel connected to them. You feel their love because they take care of you. You will be raised according to their culture, background and beliefs. They inject in you the knowledge, the knowhow and the traditions they grew up on. When you become mature and you start to explore life by all its means, you will then start to choose either to follow your guardian's lifestyle or create your own lifestyle.

Many people leave this world without knowing who they really are, because they never tried to experience something different. They never wanted to go beyond their comfort zone, and they never tried to initiate a relationship between their body, mind and soul.

They didn't know what exactly they love to do and what their system is capable of doing. Throughout their lives, they ate the same food without really knowing whether this food is welcomed by their system or not, they ate it because they were raised by their guardians, neighbors, and communities to believe that such kind of food is good and healthy for their bodies.

Many people leave this world without knowing how their bodies work, how their digestive and breathing system works or even how their muscles move. Many people didn't go the extra mile. They followed the crowd fearing the change. Their low self-esteem kept them in their comfort zone. They were so blinded by their accustomed belief. Many people have so far lived a lie and have been in denial and have been afraid to explore their true self.

They've been afraid to even communicate what they feel and what they truly believe in. Many left this world burying with them the immense doubt and fear that have shaped their entire existence. They just went by without looking within. Our body is the most powerful system created in this world.

Surprisingly enough, many people know how computers operate. They even make an effort to teach their kids about it. I wonder however if they have ever made an effort to know how their body exactly works? Have they spared some time to teach their kids about their bodies. **NO**!!! So Learn about your body and Grow Young with it.

Be DIFFERENT. Learn about **U.** Always try something new, and put yourself up for challenges to figure out how you can turn these challenges into beautiful experiences. Life is a rhyme of choices. Let therefore your intuition guide you and enjoy every choice you make. Each choice will take you somewhere new, stay tuned and enjoy the journey.

Life is a boat, be an adventurous captain. Enjoy sailing your boat and facing the high and low waves happily until you reach your last destination carrying with you beautiful experiences.

Self care is one of the areas you should prioritize in your life whether you are a male or a female, a mother or a father, single or married, a teenage or an adult. Self care is U and without loving yourself, you cannot love and take care of others genuinely. Learn how to be loyal to the U before being loyal to anyone else. When you reach your self-loyalty you can easily be loyal to others.

Many tell me, "Come on Vick" I am taking good care of my family, kids and myself… Girl, I eat and feed them healthily and I exercise from time to time. My answer is always the following.. "Helloo people, healthy and positive lifestyle is not only about eating healthy and exercising at times. Healthy and positive lifestyle is about U being in balance and sharing your happiness with others. How can you play with your kids and give them the needful care and joy, if you are tired and in bad mood and not even in harmony with your own self? How can you maintain a healthy relationship with you partner if you are deeply not accepting yourself and living an internal struggle that only you feel? How can you love your parents, relatives, and friends if you don't love yourself? How can you enjoy your work and your colleagues if you are always hot-tempered and easily irritated? How can you be in peace if you don't practice daily gratitude? How can you be at ease if you get annoyed from a taxi driver when he overtakes you in a wrong way, or shout on a waiter in a restaurant, or show attitude if they delivered your food late or not as wanted? How can you be happy if down deep you hold a grudge against people who hurt you in the past, or if the bitter past still survives within you? How? Just tell me how?". And of course, this was always enough to let them stop for seconds and ponder on these questions.

My dear reader, I want you to start prioritizing yourself and appreciating **U for a better U**. That is why I decided to write and share my stories so I can motivate you and make you see and live things in a simpler way. Healthy and positive lifestyle starts with U. Healthy and positive lifestyle is more than what you find on your plate. It is the balance between the healthy relationships, regular physical activity, a fulfilling career and a spiritual practice that will fill your soul and satisfy your hunger for life. Healthy and positive lifestyle is the bonding between you and your creator and how you practice and communicate your gratitude with the universe.

Only U Can Make U Happy, yes, it is so true, therefore start focusing on U and enjoy life positively. I never count on anyone to make me happy because I know eternal happiness lies within me. Yes, for sure we've encountered many people in our life and had people in our present life that make us happy and leave nice memories, but this joy is temporary and has an expiry date. Only your inner self can make you blissful forever. And I always emphasize that nothing is more beautiful than self confidence.

I love to share my happiness with other people who are ready to live a simple and a happy life. My religion is my daily practice which is based on self-respect, respect to others, kindness, sharing, caring, loving, giving, self-awareness, conscious acts, gratitude and most importantly honesty. My life is free from hatred, jealousy, gossip, envy, bitterness and lies. Isn't the most beautiful thing about the truth is that you don't need to remember what you actually shared with people? For that :

Live Simple - Live Happy.

Please read carefully my below tips and stories. Ignore the ones you don't agree with and the ones you like try to incorporate in your life and enjoy them.

NOW, are you ready to grow young with me, with your family, with your partner, with your relatives, friends, neighbors, colleagues, strangers. Are you ready to grow young with the whole world? The last 2 chapters are on to start and soon will finish. It took me longer time to write them due to their delicacy. I hope all my chapters will contribute to positive changes and to boosting your happiness.

The things that I will recommend for your healthy and positive transformation are very simple but need strong will, little effort, time and consistency.

1. Design Your Personalized Healthy Menu

As I mentioned in the first few chapters, the most important things in our life are to have a strong relationship with our bodies, to know every kind of food we are eating, and to choose the right nutrients that help our system to grow and nourish. Being loyal to your body makes you feel grounded. Design your own food menu and enjoy healthy eating.

When I started sharing my new nutritional consultations with my friends I felt over happy to know that they instantly changed many things in their eating habits. As a matter of fact, they started by eliminating coffee, soda, refined sugar and harmful produce from their dictionary, and what made me happier is that they shared with me their after-eating positive symptoms (They lost weight, lost fat, became toned, their skin rejuvenated, no bloating and migraine, felt more fit and energized, started to handle problems in a calmer way, etc.).

They even started to watch out more for what they are feeding their kids with. They threw all the junk foods and sweets from the house. Of course, this last thing is of crucial importance as you can't avoid the temptation of eating something if it lies there in front of you or of your kids.

They started to realize the importance of educating their kids about healthy lifestyle ever since they were young. By seeing how loyal their parents are to their bodies, they will become loyal to their bodies too.

Imagine smoking in front of your kids, will you dare to tell them not to smoke when they decide to take up smoking? The first thing they will tell you is "why are you smoking then?" Therefore, building healthy generations starts from each and every house, and starts by being the ideal models to our kids. If the majority of parents succeeded in seeding the life ethics in their kids we will for sure have a healthy world with less criminals, thieves and dangerous people.

Another thing, a lot of couples get married too young. And a lot of these couples fail at parenting only because they haven't had the chance to experience themselves stability, maturity as well as simple responsibility values. They therefore struggle to implement good values in their homes, but unfortunately fail at this. Consequently, they end up breeding ignorance and complications unwillingly. Due to this particular fact, I enjoy assisting people to take care of themselves, and I try to spread awareness to help them live better, so that they end up raising better, healthy and positive families.

I just love it when I hear and know that my words have reached some bodies. And I always tell my friends, if you guys think that being well needs high maintenance and lots of effort, try being ill and experience the difference.

2. Add Life To Your Exercise Pattern

Yes again and again, whatever your gender, age or physical condition is, you can always find time to refresh your muscles and keep them energized. Having a fit and healthy body increases your self-confidence. Start your exercise today. Do anything to remind yourself to focus on here and now, even if that means to buy some fitness accessories like dumbbells, steps and exercise while watching your favorite series at home.

Throughout my life, I have motivated many people to instigate their exercise anytime during the day; at least to consecrate 30 minutes per day for their bodies. I've invited many friends to join me for sports sessions instead of coffee gatherings. I joined them in their sports activities just to keep them motivated and I sowed the healthy seed in them.

I am delighted to hear my friends share with me their exercise stories. I love to meet people that exercise regularly, before or after their work, or anytime during the day. This means they are taking care of their muscles and appreciating their bodies. I like to see my married friends dedicating time to themselves to stay fit and sexy. Luckily I am a morning person. I love to wake up early at 5 am for a run or swim and then embark on an energetic fresh day at the office. I even like to exercise twice a day, morning and evening. I feel amazed when I come across people leading such a positive routine.

Being a sports freak, I have most of the equipments related to the sports I love to practice. Whenever I travel to a new country I have a bag full of tennis, squash and ping pong bets. In addition to hiking, cycling, spinning and swimming accessories (not to forget my underwater Ipod), bowling shoes and helmet, cycling and diving gears, speed motor biking helmet and jacket, and last but not least my nonstop sparkling energy.

Be sure, if I am going for a short vacation, you will definitely find running and swimming kits with me. I budge without them. No matter where I go, I make sure I go for a short period run or ride in the morning. This routine gives me wings to fly and explore new places, and a morning swim will keep me fresh and vibrant. Exercise always brings the little **Me in Me.**

Therefore my friend even during your vacation, try to have at least your running gears with you to enjoy a walk or a refreshing run in nature.

I did many changes to my close friends' life. For instance, some started to cycle and do spinning, others to swim, or dive. Few bought gym memberships and enrolled with personal trainers. And I just love when they tell me that whenever they feel tired and not in the mood for exercising, they remember my words and unconsciously get motivated and start their training. I always advise people to enroll their kids in different activities at a young age, even at 3 year. For instance, they can enroll them in gymnastics in order to supple their body and prepare them to do the sports they love. In fact, they will be able to excel at any sports if they have a supple body. Even swimming for kids is very essential at their very young age.

One of my swimming instructors used to have 2-month-old toddlers swimming with their parents in the pool. We need to remember that water is a familiar environment for toddlers as they were swimming in water for 9 months. And they just love the feeling. So don't think twice, trust your toddler to a certified swimming instructor in the pool and let your baby enjoy the water.

3. How Sleeping Makes Me Fresh

The human body needs around 7 to 9 hours, depending on a person's age, of uninterrupted sleep every day which will help to release the stress and boost the metabolism, the digestive system, the memory and the whole functions of the body. Sleeping is considered one of the essential life necessities. Sleeping is the only time where the body undergoes repair and detoxification.

We can never go without sleeping for more than few days. The body will be tired and soon will fall sick. Interrupted and few hours sleep promote weight gain.
I, for instance, like to sleep early and wake up early with the sunrise. And if I failed to have my 7 hours sleep, my face will on the spot burst out with pimples and I will feel down the whole day. So I make sure I compensate for the loss of sleep during the day, and have a nap. Note that each body reacts differently to sleep; so check your body and take the appropriate measures to avoid discomfort.

BUT, be careful not to exploit your sleep. Actually, oversleeping makes you tired and lowers your energy level. I have a relative we call "Mr. Sleepy", who likes to sleep a minimum of 12 hours a day. Surprisingly for a person who rests so much, he is always tired and has a lot of mood swings. It's like he's got PMS for almost the whole month. (PMS are the emotional symptoms ladies undergo before having their period). Whenever I call him, he is either sleeping or having a nap.

He is only awake during his working hours, but still I always wondered how productive he could be with that low energy he carries with him to work (specially that he works in construction and most of his work is outside in the heat). Until one day he sought my assistance and wanted to accompany me for one of my early sports sessions.

For sure, the first 10 times he failed to wake up and he missed his chance. Not until one weekend when we had a bet did he come on time. It was being on time or our friendship, as I had threatened not to talk to him anymore if he didn't join me for this particular run. Luckily he did, and we enjoyed a nice morning run and he felt refreshed throughout the day.

It wasn't easy to drag him for running especially that he was stopping and resting repeatedly, but this was expected, and still I managed to motivate him. The second day when I called to check on him and see if he was suffering from sore muscles, I was surprised to know that he had woken up early and was feeling good, and that he had gone to the gym where he had bought membership for the past 2 years but never attended.

I was overwhelmed to hear that, and since then he's accompanied me to most of my sports sessions. Plus, he lost weight, toned his muscles and above all he regained his energy. Although he still loves sleeping and is hardly managing to get by with only 9 to 10 hours of sleep, he revamped his energy and started to have control over his mood. Below are a few steps you may incorporate in your daily routine, and that will improve your sleeping patterns.

a. Meditate To Medicate

Meditation cools your system down. Therefore, if you meditate at night before you sleep, this will boost your immune system, calm you down, balance your emotions and lower your blood pressure.

I usually love to meditate in the mornings before my shower, my lemon juice and smoothies breakfast. Believe me the best thing you could offer your body and mind is meditation. Some people prefer it in the morning and others at night. If I didn't manage to practice it in the morning then the evening will serve.

Drinking a cup of lemon juice mixed with warm to hot water in the early morning, after the meditation and before breakfast, is something I would never miss. It allows me to get rid of unwanted chemicals from my body. It cleanses and energizes my whole system in the morning. Lemons are natural antiseptics and can help cure skin problems. The Vitamin C in lemons rejuvenates the skin. Moreover, drinking lemon water daily can remove wrinkles and blackheads, fade scars and reduce burning sensations to your skin. It is henceforth worth trying it. I do it to rejuvenate and wake my senses smoothly and begin a positive vibrant day.

Night meditation promotes positive mood and relaxing sleep. Even if you don't meditate, try to think of beautiful thoughts before you sleep. This generates nice feelings and pleasant dreams.

If you have never done meditation but you really want to cool your system down I will share with you few breathing techniques that you may try every morning before leaving the bed and at night before sleeping. It takes just 5 minutes from your time. Are you ready? Here we go…

Sit on your back side in your bed.
Stretch your legs forward.
Keep your back straight and your head half up.
Put your hands beside your legs, palms upwards.
Close your eyes and focus on one point between your eyes.
Disconnect from any sound around you.
Take 20 deep slow breaths and inhale deeply and exhale very slowly from your nose only.

You should be able to do it in 4 to 5 minutes. The longer the minutes it will take you the better it is. This means you are breathing slowly.

This will assist you to calm your mind down. I personally try to breath in and out from my nose most of the time because I feel more grounded, as the nose is specifically designed for breathing whereas the mouth has multi tasks.

b. Record Your Memories

Before I turn the page on my laborious day, I like to write 5 minutes about the significant incidents I encountered that same day and how they affected my decisions and mood. This reflection helps me a lot in evaluating my reactions and decisions.

After my recent relocation from Qatar to Lebanon I had enough time to fix my personal belongings and rearrange my room, where I surprisingly found my first diary. On it were those stories I wrote from the age of 14 to the age of 20.

What I found there brought forward nice memories which I had forgotten. Remembering how I used to handle my challenges at that age made me cry and smile at the same time, and I went on thinking how I would handle them now. This reflected the self - development that I have reached now. I have written about my school and university exam preparations; my personal crushes; who I used to like and how things evolved; my first salary and how I used to plan my expenses. There was also news about my sports journey with my brother and the Judo competitions we joined together; stories about my "Judo traveling".

In addition to that, there were lines about my feelings regarding my dad's cancer, and how I felt when I used to accompany him for his chemotherapy treatments and how mum used to calm me down with her motivating warm words "Dad will be ok honey, just pray for him". I found details about my painful and happy moments, and details about my success and the inconvenient things I had lived, which left me questioning why they were happening.

Of course now I understand the reasons behind all these things. And when I look back, I smile because all these mixed feelings strengthened me, made me appreciate life more, and made me who I am today. I loved the feeling of remembering Me many years ago. This motivated me more to keep on reflecting every night because I am sure one day when I reach a certain age or when the beautiful grey prevails, I will be sitting on the beach watching a beautiful sunset, reading and smiling the same way I am doing now.

Therefore, I entreat you to start writing and reflecting, not necessarily every night, you can have it on a weekly basis, but just start to reflect.

Sometimes I even reflect for 5 minutes in the very early morning when I open my eyes. I write my very first morning thoughts which mirrors my subconscious at many times. I love to plan ahead my snag list for the day to keep myself organized and set out on a beautiful day.

c. Breath Clean To Sleep Lean

I like to sleep with open windows no matter what season we are in. This is because I like to feel the fresh air circulating in my system while I am sleeping. Air-conditioning annoys me. If you like to sleep with the AC switched on, make sure to expose your house and bedroom to fresh air during the day to purify the atmosphere.

I have read many articles on the net about how central air-conditioning at home or at work can cause headaches, fatigue, mucous membrane irritation, breathing difficulties and skin irritations. Air-conditioning ventilation systems can spread contaminants in the air and pollutants such as bacteria, molds, mildew and viruses.

I don't know how accurate this information is, but what I definitely know that my system doesn't accept the air-conditioning. Even though I live in very hot countries, I try not to turn on the air-conditioner often.

d. Fresh Pores For Fresh Dreams

This is purely for my female readers. If you want to maintain a hydrated and healthy face, rule number one, remove your make up and allow your pores to breath. I remove my make - up, before I sleep, with coconut or almond oil and water (I use small face towel or cotton for that) . I like to feel that my facial skin is clean. I use virgin oils at night to hydrate my face such as coconut, olive or almond oils that will be absorbed by my skin and keep it hydrated. Even if I come late from a dinner, I make sure to clean my face for a good night sleep. Most of our makeup products are made of toxins ingredients that will harm our skin if left overnight. Wash them off well and have beautiful dreams.

e. Power Off & Sleep On

I make sure to switch off any light and electrical flow in my room before I sleep. Lights affect our sleep because of our photosensitive retinal ganglion cells that are sensitive to light. Therefore, it is better to have curtains in the room to switch off your system at night, and open the blinds in the morning to reset your system with the sun light.

We all heard and know that the flow of electromagnetic frequencies can be harmful to our system. Subsequently, any electronic device in the room affects our sleep. I know it is becoming very difficult to most of us to wake up in the middle of the night or early in the morning without being able to check our phones and see who sent us a message or an email.

BUT, we need to detox our system from the mobile effect and give space to our mind and thoughts to shut down at night and restart in the morning smoothly and positively. No one will get hurt if you don't answer their emails the minute you open your eyes, therefore don't stress your system with technology the first thing in the morning. You have the whole day to chat, answer emails and stress yourself. Try to enjoy your sleep in an electromagnetic free zone.

f. Perfect Bed & Pillow For Perfect Sleep

Always choose a nice rigid bed and a healthy pillow for your body. This will have an effect on your sleep and general comfort. I used to suffer from neck pain until I got a medical pillow which I can't sleep without now.

g. Light Stomach For Light Sleep

Don't eat late at night and sleep because when you sleep your body generates hormones that regulate growth and appetite, and if your digestive system is working this may stress your system and cause digestive problems and interrupted sleep. I am a person that doesn't like to eat and drink after 8pm in order not to have interrupted sleep.

4.Thank You Lord,Thank You Universe

The Best thing in life is to show gratitude to life. Count minimum 12 new blessings each night before you close your eyes. Say thank you for minimum 12 beautiful things or incidents that happened to you during the day and realize how many blessings you have received and have taken for granted.

We have unlimited blessings everyday to be grateful for. Be grateful for the air you are breathing, the scenery you are able to see, the sounds you are hearing, the steps you are walking, the things you are able to hold, the nice events happening around you,etc.

Gratitude will shift your focus from the unpleasant events that happened and will make you appreciate the small good things that made you smile during the day. Example, say thank you for seeing a good old friend, finding a nice parking space in the middle of a busy district, receiving nice news from your parents, your kids doing well at school, eating tasty food, your management appreciating your reports, etc, all this will generate positive and happy thoughts to your dreams.

I, for instance, always shut down my system at night with a small prayer showing gratitude for the healthy day extended to me and all the blessings that I've shared during the day, and I close my eyes wishing to have a fruitful day the next morning. We should be grateful for everything happening around us and for the life we were gifted. Keep in mind that many people don't have this privilege anymore.

Self care is my favorite ritual. I just love taking care of Me. My list can go on and on. I enjoy giving self care advice especially for working males and females, parents and singles, who don't find time to pamper themselves and prioritize everything on the account of their self. And much to their dismay, one day they suddenly wake up, look around and realize how things had passed them by, how they've missed out on the small things that they hadn't enjoyed. They wake up to realize how old they grew.

If you are a parent you should find time to take care of yourself because the healthier you are the healthier your kids become. I feel pity when I see kids at the age of 10 starting dieting or eating wrong kinds of food that will hurt them more. The poor things grow up feeling embarrassed from their bodies and in constant unsuccessful dieting processes. We are constantly learning that many kids are diabetic or are suffering from pre-diabetic conditions. We are encountering lots of overweight and obese kids. Who is responsible for this, the 5-year-old boy or his mum who kept on eating all kinds of junk food during pregnancy? Who is responsible? The 10-year-old girl or her parents who keep on feeding her with the wrong food? Who is responsible for the increase of type 2 Diabetes in societies? The unfortunate kids at school that are fed with junk food or the advertising campaigns that are bombarding every school, market place and houses? I can't help but blame parents for their lack of knowledge in feeding the incorrect food to these kids who grow fighting to reach the perfect weight, and reach their 50 and are still dieting to keep themselves healthy. Be the good model for yourself, your kids and loved ones in everything you do and in the way you think.

Many couples are suffering from the routine in their lives and my advice to them is always to take up new activities, exciting crazy plans and to make an effort to keep their love alive. For instance, plan a nice family sports day, invest in creating new surprises to each other, prioritize the relationship even if kids are around, go out for romantic dinners like old good times when you were in total love and you thought you were the only ones in Wonder Land. Why not also share what you've lived during the day. You might as well rent a nice romantic film and enjoy a serene cuddly night in front of the TV with some healthy homemade cookies. Not all good times need to be pricy.

Unfortunately, I know many couples who are divorcing, or falling into the routine cycle after a marriage that lasted for 5, 10, 15, or 20 years. This doesn't surprise me much. How can a person live peacefully with his partner if he is failing to live peacefully with his own self?

Hence, I am pretty sure that when you reconcile with the **U in U**, appreciate it and learn to love it, you'll have no trouble finding peace with your entourage or partner. Try to be a healthy and positive role model for **U**, for your kids, partner and everyone around you.

I feel annoyed when I hear my friends complaining about their partners for cheating on them. However, it is very normal for things to go wrong in the relationship when the couples are not taking good care of themselves, when they are always negative, tired and have no energy to share. Hence, they fall victims of the monotony and start looking for alternatives.

Yes, I know that there are many reasons for cheating and men and women are exposed to temptations every day, but still if you take good care of yourself and you are always fresh and energetic, you will refresh your loved ones life, add positive energy and memorable fresh activities to your journey.

Plus, when you are fit, sexy and positive, for sure you will attract your partner's attention and leave no chance for disappointment to compete with you over your happiness. Now, try to make considerable use of all the tips in this book to help you get on well with your partner.

Women have multi tasks to perform during the day especially if they are working mums. But if they don't take care of themselves, soon they will lose their partner's attention ,they will be sucked into the depression vicious cycle, and they will feel low self esteem. They might as well put on weight and feel tired, frustrated and in bad mood all the time, and soon they either push their partner away from them or they will start to search outside their home for some comfort and appreciation. (Before blaming you partner , look into yourself and make changes today, you could be the essential reason behind his attitude and actions).

There's a funny joke I always tell my friends. Two ladies met after a long time, the first one asks the other, heyyy, look at you, you have lost lots of weight? What have you done? You look gorgeous…The other one took a deep breath and replied "nothing honey, I have been in a deep depression because I caught my husband cheating on me. The former exclaimed sadly "OH, no!!!! poor you, did you divorce him? So after she smiled she said "mmmm…not yet". The other woman looked surprised and asked…not yet? How come?" And the lady in a very cool sarcastic manner replied "…naaahhh I still have 5 kg to lose."

Needless to say that men are also concerned in this topic. Hence, they need to always stay fresh, fit, nice looking, energetic and responsible active persons who bring energy to the house and not only money. They need to show their partner and kids that they are a real source of life and happiness.

They should invest their time in adding value to the marriage establishment, rather than spending their time flirting and trying to initiate other relationships with other women. Subsequently, they'll sentence their previous relationship to death while building hopes on another relationship which may not be long-lived.

On the other hand, I feel even more astounded when I hear single people saying they don't have time to exercise or are too tired or don't want to invest in the gym membership. How could they say that, no time for exercise? But they have plenty of time for Facebook and WhatsApp with nonsense topics discussing other people's lives.

They don't want to invest in exercising. Yeah, but they have money to go and have unhealthy dinners and alcohol drinks. They are tired? For sure, laziness can become a habit. You are single, and you should have plenty of time to take care of U. Honey, you are still a free bird experiencing this life alone, focus on U and add energy to your life.

Haven't you ever heard that "In life one of the 2 essential things that you cannot recover is the occasion after it is missed and time after it is gone".

I sometimes say to my single friends: "If you can't find time, how are some of our married friends finding time to take care of their bodies in spite of the loads of responsibilities they have? Some friends have 2 to 3 kids and are still managing to have a nice healthy body. You, on the other hand, are single and you are carrying with you unhealthy and disappointing figures. So move yourself and start eating healthy, kick off a good exercising routine, and be positive." I hate being harsh on my friends, but they sometimes need to be scolded.

Moving on with the self-care tips, one of my favorite tips is the spa treat, and I am sure many people agree with me.

In actual fact people go to spas to relax and disconnect form their daily routine. They may go to the spa to have a relaxing massage, a refreshing facial or simply to take care of their hair, hands and feet.

I, for example, love to go to a spa that has nice luxurious facilities where I can use the swimming pool, sauna, steam, jacuzzi and enjoy a cold plunge before my treatment. I am not a person who goes to a spa to have a quick massage or a quick facial and then go back to work and stress myself again. Personally, I am not that fan of the actual massages and facials, I enjoy the pre-massage relaxation process more.

1. Why I Love to Use Steam & Sauna

I use the sauna because it increases the blood circulation which will relieve any muscle tension, ache, pain and flash toxins from food and drink out of the body. I always take water with me to drink inside the room so I don't get dehydrated or feel dizzy. If you've never tried sauna start for 5 minutes at the first then increase the time spent there gradually.
I use steam before entering the sauna to open my skin pores because the heat and moisture combination helps in gently opening bronchial tubes leading to greater and more efficient oxygenation of the bloodstream, and in turn aiding breathing and circulation.
If you suffer from any medical condition or you are pregnant avoid using these 2 facilities.

2. Body Massage, Lovely Feeling

It is very important. It reduces the stress, anxiety and depression. Moreover, it increases blood circulation and relieves pain and stiffness. I recommend once per week a spa full body massage for those who like it and can afford it. For those of you who cannot afford spa massages for time or budget constraints, you can have your own daily massage. Rub your whole body with a small hot towel.

Try to do it every day if you can for 10 minutes after or before your sleep or shower, whenever you can. This will increase blood circulation and relaxes your muscles and gives you a nice sensation. If you want you can offer it to your partner, kids or elderly parents. It generates nice feelings. You may use few drops of essential oils, such as lavender on the towel.

3. Face Cleansing, Rejuvenating Look

Your face is the boarding pass to your inner self. You need to keep it fresh and young. Therefore book a nice facial treatment in the spa that will cleanse your pores, hydrates and lifts your skin. I recommend one facial per month for everyone. If you want to save money you can have it at home twice per month and get good results as well. You may either use luxury products for home care use, or you can blend your own natural ingredients. Improvise!

I personally used many luxurious skin products until I listened to my skin and started using home-made natural products. I know the process of blending ingredients might sound very complicated and you might not have time for it, but I recommend you to avail 15 minutes and try them once, it is fun believe me and especially when your blend succeeds and you get great results.

Ready for some tips now? Here you go...

Face Scrub: I blend baking soda, honey, coconut oil and avocado.
Face Lotion: I use natural oils such as virgin coconut, olive and almond oils. Natural virgin oils are pure and have high nutrients and antioxidant levels and are very high in electron energy. I read many books and articles about some lotions that are heated extensively causing oil to oxidize, which is not good for the skin.If you use branded skin products, read labels carefully and examine your skin regularly. The good ones might be expensive but it's worth investing. This is your face...your image.
Face Toner: I use apple cider vinegar as it regulates the PH of my skin.
Moisturizer: I use virgin natural oils (coconut, olive, almond) and aloe vera.

I am not in favor of plastic surgeries which have become a trend nowadays. I vote for healthy natural care and treatments and I enjoy my fine lines and wrinkles, as they keep on reminding me about my good experiences in life. I love to invest in nourishing my inner self to keep it young and vibrant, and this will eventually sparkle on my outer appearance. What is the use of doing botox , lifting and filling if from inside I am not in peace with myself and I am not a happy person?

These surgeries will make me happy for a certain period of time then they vanish. I have to maintain them again, whereas by being fit, happy and grateful I become equipped with eternal mind peacefulness and happiness. Yes, I do agree that some people badly need some reshaping and maintenance, but unfortunately many abused this trend and harmed their beauty instead of reshaping it. Don't get drowned in doing surgeries, instead grow young naturally.

I prevent using sun blocks on my face and body, I always wear a hat and glasses and I use natural sunscreen that prevents harmful UV rays penetrating my body. I don't use the regular sunscreens found in the market because many of them irritates my skin as they contain toxic chemicals and can harm my skin when absorbed by it. For this reason, I recommend organic products or coconut oil.

When first I heard about coconut oil as sunscreen, I was hesitant to use it, but I gave it a shot, and since then my only sunscreen is the virgin coconut oil. Coconut oil absorbs the UVA which is the good UV that our body needs and it blocks the UVB that is harmful to our skin.

If you want to use medical sunscreens make sure to learn about their ingredients before applying them to your skin. Therefore, try whichever products you find suitable and observe their reaction on your skin.

4. Hydrated Hands and Feet

This service is the highest selling service in any spa or beauty salon, as it is a need to every female and is becoming a need to males as well. Yes, you can do it at home if you want and thus save lots of money, but please do it and take care of your nails.

If you suffer from dry skin specially feet skin, try to rub your feet with any virgin oil (coconut, olive and almond), wear socks and sleep with them on. This will enhance hydration and skin repair. I use natural Aloe Vera gel as well, my favorite multifunctional plant that I've already told you about.

Some of my male friends used to make fun of those men who go to a spa for a facial, a manicure or a pedicure treatment. However, when I told them how some VIP always schedule for such treatments, they got motivated and started to schedule it as well, considering it as a privilege and a luxurious self-care treat. I love to see well-groomed people with nice trimmed nails. Therefore, when I meet a new person, the first thing I do is screen his overall look, from top to toes, as this shows how much he is cautious about his own body. And this is a red line to me. My life partner has definitely to be highly-maintained starting from his eating pattern, to exercising, to grooming and to leading a positive life.

5. Your Hair, Stylish Art

The self-care won't be complete without taking care of our hair looks. Both males and females should give lots of care to their hair, as it reflects their character and plays an essential role in leaving a good impression. We can invest in our hair in the beauty salons and we can as well prepare natural hair treatments at home.

There are many natural recipes for hair treatments. Search for some on the net or in specific books and try them to see which one fits your hair better.

Personally, I sometimes blend and use baking soda, virgin coconut oil, egg and avocado as a natural hair mask.

6. Fresh Teeth and Healthy Gum? Try Oil Pulling

I have read about oil pulling and tried it, and since then I practice it everyday. What is it about? Oil Pulling helps to clean your cavities, mouth gum and ditch any bacteria and whiten your teeth. Put one tablespoon of virgin coconut oil in your mouth and smash it for 20 minutes then spit it in the garbage, (not in the sink in order not to end up with a clogged sink.) Brush your teeth afterwards and feel the nice sensation.

It is recommended to brush our teeth after every meal to remove the food residue and to keep our breath smelling fresh and nice. I once per week as well brush my teeth with baking soda. I love the feeling afterwards. Try it as it helps to clean and whiten your teeth. Baking soda or sodium bicarbonate is a multi functional product. You can use it for many things such as removing stains from the house, for cooking and for beauty purposes. It can be also used in cleaning vegetables as it removes pesticides from them. It is a must-have product in the house along with virgin coconut oil, Apple Cider Vinegar and Aloe Vera.

7. Why and When to Shower?

Throughout the day we are exposed to many microbes and dust, and we need to wash them off ourselves. That is why shower at night is very important so we can enter our bed clean of any bacteria, fresh and have nice dreams.

I love to take my shower in the morning, in the evening, before and after exercise. It relaxes my muscles and cools me down. I love to have a hot bath after a workout or a long day. I light candles, put soft music, close my eyes and wind off my thoughts for 15 to 20 minutes. I sometimes have my fresh juice while hot bathing. Try it often, it is good for relaxation.

If I go to a dinner or any pub and expose myself to smoke or cigarettes, I make sure I take my shower and roll into my bed clean, leaving the sense of smoke away from my body and bed.

I, as well, make sure to have a shower directly after visiting the following places due to the high bacteria and microbe exposure there: airplane, cinema, taxi, metro and hospital. I make sure I don't enter my bed for a small nap with my clothes that have been exposed to these places or any place during the day.

I shower before and after entering a pool. I rinse the chlorinated pool water off my skin before exposing it to the sun to avoid any chemical reaction with my skin that might cause me skin irritation. This is very important and we should as well let our kids do it.

I love ending my warm showers with cold water as it refreshes my senses, lessens the pains in my muscles and I feel totally relaxed.

What I'd like to share with you in addition to the above is my experience with corporate executives and their self care. I have worked in the corporate world with many executive women and men, and I respect those who take care of their hygiene and their bodies. Surely, many of these executives get busy at work, and spend their time attending social events without taking care of themselves. Well the truth is, I used to get irritated in a business meeting when I saw a director, a GM or a CEO who has untrimmed nails, hair around their nose or in their ears, unshaved or half shaved, or having annoying odors.

I sometimes joked to deliver my message to them and in other times I just kept my comments for myself to avoid any embarrassment. I even felt more irritated from women executives who attended big corporate meetings wearing the same suit for a couple of days, or with improperly trimmed nails or even improperly fixed hair and bad breath or odor.

If you work in a corporate world, act as one. You need to take care of your health, figure looks, hygiene, attitude, behavior and words. I will highlight a few of these points at a later stage.

Finally, Self Care is not limited only to the skin and overall body care, but it is also extended to how and with what we cover our bodies and how we present it to the world. Therefore dress to impress is our next treat.

It is no difference if you are a man or a woman, you should always dress to feel comfortable and impress at the same time. It's a wonderful feeling when you know what suits your body and dress accordingly. It will lift your mood when you feel yourself fresh and stylish.

It is not necessary to follow the trend if the trend does not match with you. All you need to know is what color and style suits you. Be unique, have your style and walk proudly with confidence.

It is not necessary to buy expensive clothes, bags and accessories to look stylish and pretty. In millions of occasions I encountered wealthy and famous ladies wearing the most expensive clothes and accessories that unfortunately don't match with their style. It is nice to wear branded clothes if you can afford them, but most importantly is to cover your body with appropriate clothes that suit you.

Love your body and appreciate every single part in it, and whatever you wear, will just shine on you. Moreover, be comfortable with what you are wearing. Don't leave the house if you are not comfortable with the clothes or shoes you are wearing because you will remain uncomfortable the whole day or night. Many people wear tight clothes or very high heels and suffer the whole day. They don't realize that annoying shoes or uncomfortable clothes may affect their mood, spoil their day, in addition to preventing their blood from circulating freely inside their veins.

Now, if you think you are bored with your style or need a new look, you can hire a professional image consultant who can advise you with many looks that suit you.

It is nice to ask your partner, parents or friends, about how you look in this dress, outfit, or suit. It will make them feel happy to know you are taking their advice, and happier that their personal opinion matters to you especially if you were asking your partner. They will feel nice and this will tighten the bonding.

Nevertheless, I repeat again and again: your body might react differently to things that are causing comfort to me or to others. Try U and listen to your own U.

" U and only U, knows exactly what suits U & makes U happy. "

Chapter Eight

■ Joy To The Soul

The final pages of my healthy journey as well as the tips to yours unfold in this chapter. Chapter 8. Eight, my lucky number as I was born on 8-8-1978. By now you've learnt a lot about who I am, about my healthy transformations. You've read my diversified recommendations about staying fit and healthy and now it is the time to share with you the reasons why I am always on the moon as my family and close friends tell me.

They always tell me, how can you do this? How can you stay calm and handle all this pressure with smiles? How can you forgive people who hurt you that easily? How can you not feel irritated form anything? Do you fear confronting people or situations? And they keep on wondering what is behind my positive attitude towards life. As a matter of fact, the real reasons behind my attitude is Me and only Me. It is how I perceive things from a different angle; the angle that reflects positive images to my eyes and maintain my positive vibes spinning.

There is a big difference between wanting to change something and willing to change it. Almost everyone wants to change things in their lives to become better and happier. However, only, and I repeat only very few take the initiative and come out from their comfort zone to try something new, face their challenges and change what they want for a better life.

Therefore, be from the many who are willing to make these changes and not just pray and wait for miracles to happen. Miracles lie in the very core of your own self and your own decisions. So make them happen. Attract only the positive vibes towards your life from the energy that exits everywhere around us.

Keep in mind that **"a journey of a thousand miles begins with a single step"** Laozi. Therefore,take baby steps as "it is better to take many small steps in the right direction than to make a great leap forward only to stumble backward."Change little things in your life first and soon everything starts to fall into place.

A specific incident or situation may inflict pain upon us. And yet,since suffering is only a state of mind, decide yourself whether you want to live it or not. Decide whether you want to be from those who give way to tragedy and keep on whining, thus allure more misery, or from those who move on and don't let life's bumps cloud their lives. Don't wait until you are lying there in that hospital bed, helpless and almost lifeless, to look back and wish you had changed or lived better. Mark the first milestone on the pathway of your rejuvenation.

You need to find the balance in your life to live a healthy and a positive one. Therefore you should take care of your body, your soul as well as your mind.

"It is good to have an end to a journey towards, but it is the journey that matters, in the end" - Ursula Guin. Depending on your definition of success, the difficulty of your journey will differ too. If money and public success are what matter to you the most, you are likely to have a hard time along your life path.

You don't want to reach your 90 years suffering from all kind of stress, diseases and waiting for your final moment to arrive. I want you to reach your 90 with lots of hopes and plans and a wish to accomplish them.

And now that you've become equipped with tips for a healthier body, take a little more time to read the following pieces of advice.

Love of Arts Is A Soul Nutrient

Many people I know enjoy different kinds of arts to pamper their souls. For instance, many friends like to play music when they have free time. They initiate a bonding with musical instrument that reaches their souls and soothes their mood. Some, on the other hand, listen to their favorite music which in turn cools them down and unwinds them from their surroundings.

Others vent their stress by feeding their souls with the act of painting beautiful works of art, and feeling happy while closing their eyes and letting their thoughts flow with the brush.

Singing is another way that many people enjoy to shift their mood. Dancing is also refreshing. I saw people distressing and swinging their bodies in a healthy and joyful way.

Why don't you then try to experience these different kinds of arts and listen to the comfort of your soul? Indulge in finding the most suitable way to vent your daily stress. I, for example, never thought writing is my retreat until I tried it at the age of 36. Hence, the more you know about yourself, the more comfortable you will feel and less incidents will win over your good mood.

Improve Your Knowledge

Many people feed their souls by reading books and by enriching their knowledge. Others, however, think academic learning stops after they receive their university degree. I renounce this idea because I strongly believe that people will enjoy learning when they're older more than they enjoy it when they were teenagers. When they're older, they do it voluntarily whereas at school and university they considered learning as a burden or a punishment. How many young have enrolled in majors they thought they'd love, and realized it wasn't what they had wanted only after they start working? Then, they wish they had chosen another major. At a certain mature age and after experiencing the real life and the corporate world, many people I know continued their studies and chose majors that fit their passion more.

I love to enroll in short and long periodic courses to enhance my knowledge. These cources enlightened me to write my first book... which I am in the many courses i have enrolled in enlightened me write my first book enlightened me to write my first book, which I am in love with. I put so much positive energy in every letter I wrote, and I won't stop here as I am planning to write more books related to different aspects of life.

I as well want to learn more than the 4 languages I already know (Arabic, Armenian English and French) and get more diplomas in diversified fields. There is no such thing as a suitable age for learning. I feel inspired by seeing 50 years and older people attending universities or institutes to continue their studies. Find time, set a budget, and learn a new language or enroll in a course you like. Believe me you will feel content, refreshed, more knowledgeable and proud of U when you receive your diploma or degree.

Allow Others' Souls to Feed Your Soul

I love volunteering in charity organizations and helping kids with special abilities (as I like to call them), as well as elderly and needful people. In fact, in every country where I've resided I used to search and enroll directly in such organizations and devote time despite my busy work schedule to assist them. I feel alive by contributing my energy to sparkling their souls.

I actually dedicate one trip per year to travel with charity organizations to different countries to assist needful kids and communities. And I let my energy flow throughout the trip among these people, where my smiles are multiplied freely and my soul sings joyfully. I learn a lot from every person I meet in these trips. They teach me how to appreciate life more and feel grounded.

Once, in one of the art charity events, while I was pushing a kid on his wheelchair and playing around with him, he saw a girl drawing a beautiful forest on the foam boards. He felt excited to ask her about her drawing, but she couldn't hear him. At that point, he noticed that she was deaf and couldn't speak. He felt bad for her. She saw the sadness in his eyes and then approached to kiss him. At the same time, she was gesturing to explain to him something. When she finished her assistant looked at the boy sitting on his wheel chair and told him " honey, she is telling you not to be sad because she cannot hear or talk to you. She promises you that one day you will both meet somewhere very beautiful where she will be able to talk and hear and you will be able to walk". When I heard this sentence, my whole senses froze except for my eyes, which were filled with tears. I asked the assistance to hold the wheelchair for me and I ran to a nearby corner and released my tears silently as I didn't want anyone to see me crying especially the little boy and girl.

There I felt overwhelmed at the thought of being a healthy person with no disability whatsoever; and I felt the pure heart and the inspiring souls these kids have. It is ironic how the special abilities these kids possess never go unnoticed, while our world is full of people with mental hidden disabilities that are only perceived when we are in direct contact with them whether at work or in social gatherings. And unfortunately, these disabilities, those persons walk with, hurt other people and ruin families and societies.

The abilities of these special kids are engraved in my mind. If sometimes I feel unable to laugh, or if I encounter a difficulty in accomplishing a task, I remember one of them and I feel inspired. Moreover, their memories bring energy to my senses.

So my dear reader, embrace this advice from me please find time to contribute to such associations because giving and sharing is a blessing. Of course you can contribute financially, but when you initiate direct contact with them you will be reciprocally contributing to nourishing your soul with all the positivity anyone needs. One hour per week from your precious time can make a needful soul happy and you will draw a smile on beautiful faces.

Do it and feel the positive impact on you. Never say that you cannot handle the situation, yes it is a bit challenging but the outcome will be quite empowering to you. You will learn how to appreciate your life challenges more.

One of the challenging things that I would like to highlight in this chapter is the positive thoughts that we need to keep on embracing, and which have a direct impact on our daily interaction with our parents, partners, kids, friends, colleagues, neighbors, strangers and the world in general.

Sometimes we look at our life and say "Oh I can't do this, or I can't do that. It's too hard for me. Other times we look at people who are in our life and we say "Oh, I really can't stand this person anymore". Sometimes we nag about what we have and envy what others have "Oh, I wish I had more money so I can stop working and have a relaxing life like my neighbour". Many other times we say "Ufff, I wish I had a better job and nicer colleagues", or "Wawooo…I love her body, I wish I had one like it ". Some single people might wonder why they're still single "When am I going to meet Mr. Right everyone is getting married?". Married will say "mmmmm, I wish I was still single and free of all this family hassle and could enjoy my time alone". And we keep on concentrating on the things we wish to have or things we wish we didn't have and we forget about what we do have.

Unfortunately, by doing so the current moments fly us by leaving behind the joy we could have had through living them. We do that often, and forget that we can't return back in time.

In life there are key principles, one of which is to learn how to be grateful for everything we have and have achieved. We need to learn how to be grateful for having a life while others were banned from this privilege. In truth, it's a big lie to think that you are not good. It's a big lie to think that you're worth nothing. You ought to love yourself, love your body, love your abilities in life.

A resounding Yes, Yes, Yes…Yes, I know it's sometimes difficult to smile in life when undesired events happen and we don't know why, and we don't know if we will outlive them. Yes, it's not easy to go through our storms and we don't know how long the storms are staying. But one thing we should learn, and it is how to be patient.

It is very strange to see people with eating and sleeping disorders and bad relationships with their family, parents, friends and colleagues. It's a pity how many people suffer from inferiority and feel they're worth nothing when they have everything. And on the other hand, it is a blessing to see people having fewer abilities and fewer blessings and are content with what they have.

Each one has to look within, to look at the beauty that lies there and try to share it with the world. Ponder for instance on that: How many unhappy rich people do you know? How many unhappy celebrities do you hear about? How many unhappy beautiful ladies and gents do you encounter in your life? How many unhappy slim, sexy and fit people do you meet daily? How many unhappy successful business people do you know? Don't you question all these divorces and cheating happening around, when for some time you thought these people were experiencing happy relationships and had lovely families?

Imagine for a minute that you'd lost an organ, such as an eye, hand, leg, or arm. What importance would being rich, successful, skinny, beautiful, etc. have? Will all the latter mentioned be of any value? Wouldn't you just wished you had all your organs and could start new?

When was the last time you did something new and came out of your comfort zone? When was the last time you spent consecutive 10 happy days without any disappointment or anger? Come on…try something new, face your fears, challenge yourself and see what you are capable of handling. Life is fun…life is an adventure… smile more often…help others regularly and most importantly…
Enjoy U being U.

Therefore, do never think that any achievement you make in your life is more powerful than the bond you initiate between U and Your Own Body, Mind and Soul. Bear this in mind: **Only U can change U**.

As a matter of fact, this feeling gives me positivity throughout the day, and helps me to control my reactions towards any incident that happens to me at work or on a personal level. I manage well to keep my positive vibes dominate, and I feel bad if anyone managed to win over me and bring my negative vibes on.

How many of us have encountered twitchy colleagues who've had a negative impact on our day. How many of us have had contact with peers' negative vibes. Indeed, at work we communicate with different colleagues and clients who have different lifestyles. For example, some are facing many problems in their personal life and are carrying it to work. Their attitude and behavior is often full of hatred, complications and is overloaded with negative energy that they willingly want to spread all over the place. I call these types of people **"Mr. & Mrs. Attitude"** Indeed, I do get annoyed by their attitude, but I manage smartly to keep their bad energy away from my positive zone.

I don't fire back with the same weapon. I try however to release my positive thoughts through understanding their reaction and understanding the reason behind their attitude. Instead of facing them in the same way they are communicating, I try to cool them down. Then in a calm way I deliver my message to them, explaining that I was annoyed from their behavior. You'll be surprised to learn that most of the time, I make them feel sorry and appreciative of my patience.

A lot of friends always voice their concern about being nice to their colleagues. They fear being taken for granted, which unquestionably often happens. My answer is always: "be yourself, considerate, level-headed, and helpful and don't mind others." I am not denying the fact that the corporate world can be like a living jungle where almost everyone is as sly as a fox.

Moreover, I can't renounce the fact that working these days has become like an episode of "Survival"…everyone is willing to go to extremes in order to attain his personal gains. But, that doesn't necessarily mean that you should lose your integrity in order to go with the flow.

Like you I've had my share of such people. I even came to a point of distinguishing them immediately at first or second encounter. It is like their behavior permeates the office.

Who doesn't know **"Miss Skirty"** or **"Miss Bra"** the one who is ready to initiate any intimate relationship with the boss and executive colleagues to reach her goals. She is "the untouchable employee" everyone gossips about, and yet stay on good terms with her. Unfortunately, in many cases these people lose their positions as fast as the wind as the new collection or the new joiners might compete against them.

You will always find **Mr. & Mrs. Show Off** who always want to be seen by everyone and would like their work to be acknowledged even if it is on the expense of their peers. These people just make me laugh.

There is also **Mr. & Mrs. "I Know Everything"**, who surprisingly have an answer to anything and never fail to impose their opinions on everyone around."Do they know we know they don't know?" Hilarious!!!! No!!!!!

"Mr. & Mrs. Polish" Best performance rewards go to them for their leading roles at deceiving others by all possible means. They are the managers' St Patrick's dog and colleagues' living hell.

Mr. & Mrs "BS", the back stabbers who instead of investing their time doing work they just plan on how to undermine their colleagues so they can shine. These people can come in handy with gangsters as to give a hand in planning destructive schemes.

Last but not least **"Mr. & Mrs. Sneaky"** the ones who like to show sweetness to the new employees and gossip about other colleagues to win their friendship. Give them a story and get in return a movie.

The boss, being a successful person, must know all these scenarios Therefore if you are honest, respectful and confident person, you will win his genuine trust. Just focus on your work without minding the artificial people.

Be Different...Be U.

I always say, that any monster you encounter in your life was once a cute small baby full of sweetness and was loved by everyone. But life's challenges and his chosen choices made him who he is today. For this, try to reach the good in this person by reflecting who you really are from inside. As far as I am concerned, I have learnt throughout the years how to control my words, and how to utter the instructive ones only.

To tell the truth, if any small or big incident happened to me, I try automatically to cool myself down, boost my positive thoughts, translate the matter in a positive way and go on with my day.

For example, I was once in a restaurant where I was having lunch with my friend. After we placed the order, it came a bit different. She was furious, beckoned the waiter and gave him a piece of her mind. Things didn't stop here. She texted her partner and her negativity pervaded his day. I, on the other hand, continued enjoying my meal peacefully. And when she finally came to her senses we had a small chat about the incident. She realized how unnecessary all this scene was and apologized to the persons concerned.

Whenever you find yourself in a similar situation and things are starting to get out of hand, step back for a second and remember how fortunate you are to be enjoying a meal while many others are dying to satiate their hunger with bread crumbs.

My dear reader, we get stressed over many unimportant things in life and we invest so much negative energy in them. Moreover, we change our mood, and we annoy our surroundings with nonsense things. Believe me negative energy attracts negative energy and positive energy attracts positive energy. So stay positive no matter what is happening around you and be sure positive outcome will come your way.

When it comes to me, I try hard not to let anything affect the peace and serenity I live. There is however only one thing that paralyses my positive thoughts and makes me feel devastated. It is when someone dear to me dies, and yet also then I suppose we all should be grateful for having had this person in our life even for a short period of time. We should be grateful because many people were not blessed to have a dear person like him/her in their lives.

Another vital thing, I wish you would accomplish, is to understand and accept the others and try to help those who seek help silently. Despite the fact that this theory seems difficult to achieve, it is worth trying it for your sake first and for others' sake second.

This actually was a theory I had to forcefully embrace and make others embrace after a twisted and degraded thing occurred to me. One time at work an executive from one of the affiliated companies spread a rumor about me in the purpose of hurting me. It didn't take me long to decide how to handle the situation with righteousness, confidence and niceness. How?

To start, my management, who knew me well and of course trusted my integrity, supported me 100%. This is something I will never forget: how my employer and his family, management and colleagues stood by me. I was lucky at many times during my career to have worked with respectful, genuine and professional employers, who've considered me as a member of their family.

This executive sick person left the company few weeks before this incident because the management had caught him abusing his executive position and as a matter of fact the management sought my assistance to provide some evidence related to his misbehavior. Apparently he thought that I was the one who initiated the investigation and he wanted to avenge.

To overcome the inconvenient feeling this rumor had generated in me, I spent a while praying for this person and wishing that his soul would be cleansed from the sick mentality and ugly feelings that have been rooted in him for years, and which made him the disrespectful sick person he has turned out to be. Moreover, I turned down any attempt of talking about the subject from the other colleagues who wanted to show their support to me.

Because as I mentioned earlier, once this monster was a beautiful innocent little soul but his lifestyle and greediness, and maybe the need to thrive made him become the bad person he is now. My colleagues wondered how I could think like this and my answer was "I learnt how to forgive in order to heal myself, and how to let go in order to grow young".

I am sure many of you have faced or heard similar incidents, because the world is full of bad spirits. The corporate world can be so cruel. My advice to you my friend is not to focus on such materialistic actions and thoughts.

However, enjoy your work positively; communicate with your colleagues with respect while enjoying a balance between work, family and self-care. Invest in your own happiness with gratitude. How many times did you change work thinking you will find your dream job and a nicer atmosphere and surprisingly you enter into the viscous circle again where you have fights with your management, colleagues and want to look for another job again? This is life. It is not about the others it is about U and how U handle the others positively and nicely by reflecting the real clean you.

Learn how to love what you are doing or do what you love. In both cases learn to live life with evolvement and good intentions never with attachments and expectations that lead to disappointments which will hurt your soul.

I always try to motivate people with my stories and how I have dealt with them. I love spreading motivational and positive thoughts wherever I go. I strongly believe someone's nice words might fill an empty place in someone's heart and someone's care might fill an empty space in someone's life.

Once I was chosen by one of the International women's associations where I was a team leader, to join a mentor and mentee program (it is a program where the mentor advises and assists his/her mentee to develop some of his/her skills). My mentee was a 38-year-old South African married woman who is a wine specialist but was working as a PA in one of the companies.

During our first meetings she informed me that she was unhappy with her job and that it's been 4 years she's pursuing it. She added that she didn't know what to do. As you may know me well by know, you must have guessed that I started to inspire her to either find ways to accept and love her current job or to find a more appropriate job where she can enjoy her passion. Every time we meet I used to tell her "Honey, you are not a tree, move from your comfort zone. Don't let your fear be your pilot. Start searching for an alternative job or just learn to enjoy what you are doing with gratitude.

Every time I encountered her I used to give her examples about how I left from one job to another, what I did, how I managed and so on. After a month from the program, she called me screaming…" Vixxx, guess what? I found my dream job and I am resigning tomorrow," I was speechless and over happy. Speechless because I knew that the persistence and the positive energy she's put in finding a job helped her to find her dream job. She joined a luxurious hotel as a wine specialist director in charge of all its restaurants. How charming, heartwarming and enticing is this.

Few weeks later, I visited her with my friends and when she saw me she approached our table and with a loud vibrant voice she told my friends." Do you see my big smile? This lady is behind it" she brought tears to my eyes with her words and with seeing her wearing her corporate suit and enjoying what she was doing. She put so much love in her job and was enjoying every bit of it.
I always tell my friends, I don't work, I practice my hobby and the minute I feel I am working I will start looking for another job where my passion can be conveyed and love can be permeated in everything said and done.

Now, finally we reached the part I like you to read and be inspired by. I will share with you 3 motivational stories, one about my kidnapping experience and that is a hell of a story, one about my dad's cancer survival journey and the last one is about my lovely British friend Darren who's inspired me with his strong will and astonishing story. And I promised to share his story with the world because I strongly believe it can change the lives of many people who are suffering out there from overweight, obesity and type 2 Diabetes.

My Kidnapping Trial

On 7th of August 2005, one day before my birthday, I was returning home at 3am from a friends' gathering with my dear old best friends for 20 years, Elie and Nadine Waked. Suddenly a car stopped in the middle of a dark street and 5 armed men started running towards our car. I was sitting in the front seat next to Elie who was driving. The minute we saw them coming, Elie tried to call the police but they had reached us before and opened the car, pushed me out of it and started to beat Elie on his head with a gun to take the phone away from him.

At that moment, I managed to run and escape while listening to the voice of Nadine shouting, "Please don't kill my only brother". While I was fleeing, I reached to a point where I couldn't hear Nadine's voice anymore. At that point I felt like if a superior power told me to stop and look back.

When I did, I saw a man with his raffle pointing at me to shoot. It was the worst feeling I have ever experienced and for the first time in my life I was crying so deeply and loudly and I begged him not to kill me stating that I will come towards him. Fortunately, he didn't shoot me. He dragged me by my hair to the car where my 2 friends were lying with the guns in their heads, and then the kidnapping journey started. They kidnapped us for about 6 hours.

The reason behind it was to steal Elie's brand new car, the Hummer H2. They drove us to very deserted places where the 3 of us experienced the worst feelings ever. We started imagining the worst scenarios, from being raped, to being rolled down the bushes, or being shot. Fortunately none of this happened, but we were at stake by just being around these criminals. To make this long adventurous story short, they released us and we faced some dangerous challenges until we reached home safely.

Every year, one day before my birthday we remember this frightful incident and I always say I was reborn that day, as at that moment we thought that we will not live again. That is why whatever challenges I face in my life now, I always refer to this kidnapping incident and tell myself " Hey girl, you were about to be murdered, and yet survived, cheer up and enjoy life". We can lose our precious life in seconds and lose everything we have.

Then try not to be consumed with this world's trivial things and enjoy being alive. Do not be like those unfortunate materialistic people who love to enjoy the artificial life and feel happy to belong to show off societies ignoring the essence of the real simple life. Do not worry over nonsense things. Do not ignore the most important things. Do not ignore your own self and own respect.

Pipo and Life

My Dad Pierre, whom I like to call Pipo, was diagnosed with chronic depression at the age of 26. He suffered from depression due to the incidents that he had lived during the war in Lebanon. Our house was bombarded and Pipo had to save many people while watching many others die which forced him to stay at home for many years.

Doctors were treating him with multi medications until he was diagnosed by the thyroid cancer at the age of 40 and he underwent chemotherapy treatments. He lost his hair, some of his teeth and lost lots of weight.

He was struggling with death, but his positive spirit and my mum's strong presence in his life lift him up. She cooked healthy food which is suitable for his body. (Lots of fruits, vegetables, meat and fish.) She also managed to provide him with as much as comfort inside the house, and poured so much love in everything she did to alleviate his depression.

Despite its downsides, my dad's sickness made me stronger and more positive. I've managed since then to look at life in a simpler way, to appreciate the small things and to enjoy life with all its ups and downs. I've learnt to watch out for my health from a young age and believe in healthy living.

At that time Cancer was barely heard of and people used to think it is a contagious disease. Many relatives and friends avoided visiting us fearing that they will catch the disease. There wasn't sufficient awareness in this regard, but in spite of all the environmental aspects, we as a family stood by our dad, cheered him up, pampered him and lifted his spirits. Moreover, we successfully beat this fatal disease and we saved our dad.

Now he is 64 years and completely cured, and yet has periodical medical checkups. He hasn't given up on smoking although he's quit alcohol. This means I still have a challenge to make him quit smoking like I did with mum.

Many factors helped stimulate my father's cancer. As a matter of fact, he used to be a heavy smoker and used to drink alcohol. What is more, he used to prefer fried food. He was under many medications and had to see different doctors who were trying to help him overcome his depression.

When my dad was diagnosed with cancer, another classmate's father was diagnosed with blood cancer at the same time too. And in that particular year we had the official academic exams of grade 9 to submit (in Lebanon we sit for an official national exam both in grade 9 and 12, according to which we either pass a class or not). What happened is that my dad recovered and I succeeded my exam whereas unfortunately her dad died and she failed the exam. I cried a lot when I knew about her dad and since then and up to this moment and for the rest of my life I will always be grateful for what happened to me, and I will always be blessed to have my Pipo around me.

In spite of his chronic depression, I was grateful that he is in good health; he can walk, talk and is managing to live a relatively normal life within the four walls of the house. To keep myself in balance and positive I always believed that one day he will regain his power and he will come back to live a normal life outside the house. I used always to think that many people have paralyzed dads in the house, or dads suffering from critical medical conditions and many lost their dads or did not even have the privilege to be raised by one. All these positive thoughts kept me going on and made me a stronger and a more responsible young girl who's known how to take care of her family with a big appreciative smile on her face, since a very young age.

Luckily there was a miraculous (if I may call it so) turning point to my dad's long lived depression. It all happened 5 years back, when I bought my own house.

When the house was ready I came to Lebanon to celebrate my birthday with my friends and I did a housewarming dinner. What is more, I refused to take one single little step in the new house without the presence of Pipo. At the beginning, he refused and said he couldn't go adding that he would be suffocated in the traffic while driving, and he would lose control and balance. In short, he insisted that he was not ready, and was weak. All these alibis were being thrown at my mum's face and mine as well. Not until several motivational tries and talks from mum and me, did we manage to pull the 49-year-old man out of his prison where he had voluntarily spent 33 years of his life.
That was the biggest achievement I had ever done in my whole life, to an extent that no one believed what was happening. No one believed that dad had been pulled out of his depression and started to live again.
It was a fulfilling and extraordinary challenge to give a life again to a 49-year-old man... my Pipo.

I love you pipo and I am glad that I started to enjoy life more with you outside the house and go on family trips all together, trips that were always like a dream to me.

When I ask Pipo how he feels if he looks 33 years back, he tells me one thing "I regret my choice that made me waste my golden years struggling with myself. Depression is not a part of our life it is our inability to manage our system. We create stress and live depression in our thoughts. Depression is not about this job or this person, or any particular incident. Depression is the offspring of our own minds, raised by our own will and nurtured by our own choices."

Pipo's story is one of its kind and I love to share it with unlimited smiles although it is painted with many unpleasant moments.

And now let us check Darren's story.

Darren Danks, one of my friends whom I've met while studying at IIN, was generous enough to give me the chance to report his exceptional turnover story from being the fat boy who was suffering from Type 2 Diabetes to the fit and slim New Darren. He lived to eat and now he eats to live. Please check his story and get inspired.

"Hi I'm Darren and I'm an ex fatty and type 2 diabetic. "Ex?" I hear you say? Well yes, you see I used to be overweight, had type 2 diabetes, high cholesterol, and high blood pressure. I used to feel shy, embarrassed, and unhappy with my body and figures. All my clothes were baggy and loose, so that no one could see how fat I really was. I'd been fat all of my life and when I reached the ripe old age of 41, I came across a movie called "Hungry For Change". Now this wasn't one of those AHH-HAA moments when I watched it. In fact, angels didn't begin to sing and harps didn't start playing. I actually thought "let's give it a go, see what happens", and so midway through September 2012 (Friday 14 September to be precise) I decided to eliminate virtually all processed foods from my diet, all coffee (I used to be a 4-5 buckets of coffee guy), all white refined foods (sugar, flour, rice), all dairy, and at that time all red meat. I wanted to start juicing after seeing Jason Vale in the movie, but not having a juicer at that time, I started making green smoothies for my breakfast.

I had a salad for lunch and a healthy meal in the evening. After a day or two I hit the detox wall and had the headaches for 3 days as my body started to remove the toxins. I started seeing weight results within a week or two and this pushed me to pursue this lifestyle.

After around 2 months, as my meat and fish intake was naturally reducing, I decided to go fully on a plant-based diet. By that time I'd changed over from smoothies to juicing and I was seeing some really good weight loss results. I was also feeling better than I had been feeling for a long, long time!

Fast forward to March 2013 when I had to have my yearly diabetic blood test. My fasting blood sugar went from 8.5 mmol/l (153mg/dl) with medication before I started this journey to 4.8 mmol/l (86.4 mg/dl); my blood pressure went from too high to normal, and my cholesterol went from too high with medication to being at the low end of the normal range. 3 months later, I had to have another blood test to confirm the March results, and my fasting blood sugar level had dropped down to 4.4 mmol/l (79 mg/dl). That was in June 2013. And at the beginning of that year, I stopped taking ALL the medications for diabetes, cholesterol and blood pressure. I just didn't need them although I can't recommend doing that without medical advice.

So in short, I cut out processed foods, and refined foods. I also changed over to fresh fruit and vegetables and I changed my life completely, lost 95lbs (43kg) and now feel amazing!"

How can I hear such a motivational account and be greedy enough not to share it with you, not to show you that impossible is only a theory, and not to give you hope that you too can be another Darren.

❝ Take care of your body and keep on growing healthier together again ❞

Congratulations...

U're a New U. Chances are you've started to clean the mess in your fridge and if not, take a moment to acknowledge that you are one step away from becoming the long desired U.

I do hope you have enjoyed reading about my experiences, and my stories have inspired you and motivated you to look deep into your life and appreciate every part of your body, soul and mind.

Finally, if you'd like to know: I enjoyed motivating Darren to start running and to participate in the upcoming UK Marathon and I am sure he will do just great. I also put Pipo on an exercise program and little by little he is going to become an energetic exerciser.

You may find the pictures of most of my stories on my website, have fun. If you need any specific further details please send me an email on the below link.

www.zestylifestylez.com

I would lastly like to narrate to you one of my favorite stories by Loren Eiseley that made a difference in my life, **"The Starfish Story"**.

"Once upon a time, there was a wise man who used to go to the ocean to do his writing. He had a habit of walking on the beach before he began his work.
One day, as he was walking along the shore, he looked down the beach and saw a human figure moving like a dancer. He smiled to himself at the thought of someone who would dance to the day, and so, he walked faster to catch up. As he got closer, he noticed that the figure was that of a young woman, and that what she was doing was not dancing at all.

The young woman was reaching down to the shore, picking up small objects, and throwing them into the ocean. He came closer still and called out «Good morning! May I ask what it is that you are doing?». The young woman paused, looked up, and replied «Throwing starfish into the ocean». «I must ask, then, why are you throwing starfish into the ocean?» asked the somewhat startled wise man. To this, the young woman replied, «The sun is up and the tide is going out. If I don't throw them in, they'll die». Upon hearing this, the wise man commented, «But, young lady, do you not realize that there are miles and miles of beach and there are starfish all along every mile?

You can't possibly make a difference!» At this, the young woman bent down, picked up yet another starfish, and threw it into the ocean. As it met the water, she said, «I made a difference to that one!"
This story reflects the power within each one of us to make a real difference to our businesses, teams, families, friends, colleagues, communities and the lives of others.

It is a powerful reminder that we can support other people by helping them to stay healthy, and lead positive lifestyles to reach their goals. It is a reminder to support them to become successful and fulfill their needs.
The starfish story is all about making a difference to the world in which we live. The Starfish is all about putting all our forces together to attain that difference and the question we ask is "What difference have you made today, to U, to your life, your family, your friends, your community or to the life of someone else?"

Do you think my book made a difference ❓

With Love and Gratitude

Victory Assaf

Lifestyle Consultant / Motivational Speaker / Author

Recepies

Check my below website link and benefit from more than 50 different kinds of simple yummy delicious recipes....Enjoy it :)

www.zestylifestylez.com

References

To enjoy more reading please visit the below links

Bio Individuality, Blood Type, Statistics and lots of Nutrition information:
www.integrativenutrition.com

Functional Medicine:
www.functionalmedicine.com

Benefits of Green Vegetable, Sweet Vegetable and Fruits:
www.integrativenutrition.com;
www.nutrition-and-you.com/vegetable-nutrition.html

Definitions:Gluten Free,Refined Sugar, Natural Sugar,Lactose Intolerant,Processed Food,Organic, Conventional Food,GMO, Nutrients:
www.integrativenutrition.com; www.livescience.com

6 essential nutrients:
www.foodpyramid.com/6-essential-nutrients
www.nutritional-supplements-information.com/list-all-vitamins.html
www.organicfacts.net/health-benefits/minerals/minerals.html

Benefits of Water:
www.integrativenutritio.comhttp://people.chem.duke.edu/~jds/cruise_chem/water/watdiet. html];
www.foodpyramid.com/6-essential-nutrients/

Healthy and Non Healthy Processed Food:
www.integrativenutrition.com;
www.epyk.com/192/7-most-unhealthy-processed-foods-you-need-to-avoid/;
www.medical-dictionary.thefreedictionary.com

Caffein:
nih.gov

Definitions: PMS, Triathlon, Aerobic, Anaerobic, Metabolism
www.medical-dictionary.thefreedictionary.com

Digestive System
www.biology.about.com/od/organsystems/a/aa032107a.htm

Muscles:
www.livestrong.com/article/88742-three-types-muscles-human-body/

Breathing:
www.breathing.com/articles/benefits.htm

Elephant Symbol:
www.shamanicjourney.com/article/6034/elephant-power-animal-symbol-of-commitment-royalty-strength